Table of Contents

1. Where Are The Glory Calls?

The telephone rings and four pair of feet jump into action. The first pair heads for the TV to lower the volume while pair #2 races to open the garage doors. Pair #3 makes a beeline for the telephone while the last pair circles around to the extension phone so not a word is lost.

It isn't a typical response to a telephone call, but it's not supposed to be. This is an ambulance station.

The message coming over the phone line is also not typical. The caller is fighting to maintain self-control as she relays her message. Her husband hasn't been feeling well and he suddenly fell to the floor unconscious. She thinks he's dead.

In moments we're racing to the scene with lights flashing and siren wailing. A thousand thoughts are going through my mind. What equipment will I need to bring in with me – will that truck approaching the intersection yield the right of way? Who am I working with tonight? A quick glance reminds me. I've got a rookie, fresh out of EMT (emergency medical technician) school. This is only his third shift. It's his first shift with me. This call will require the strong leadership approach. I brace myself.

Ten minutes later our "patient" is signing a refusal of service form. A week-long flu had resulted in a momentary fainting spell. He's telling us in no uncertain terms that he's not interested in any damn ambulance ride. His threatening eyes foretell the verbal lashing his wife will receive for subjecting him to this embarrassment. Under different circumstance her quick action might have saved his life – but this fact is lost in the anger of the moment.

"Is this the only action you guys ever get?" asks Randy Whitman on the way back to the station. "All I've had is refusals and bullshit calls since I've started here. Where are the glory calls?"

I just smile. There's no way to explain, but his misconception won't last long.

Four months later it's Randy jumping for the phone. As I study his face on the way to the call of a "sick woman" it's hard to believe this is the same rookie. He's come a long way. The nervous twitch and tension are gone. Randy's calm, in control and looking good – too good.

As we enter the house we hear a panic-stricken voice crying, "I'm dying, I'm going to die."

One step inside the bedroom is enough to confirm my worst fears. Our patient is cyanotic and mottled. She's leaning forward in her chair gasping for air and her eyes are wide with fear.

I've seen this type of patient about one hundred times which is one hundred times too many. You get a sinking feeling in the pit of your stomach that no matter what you do this patient is going to die. You get that feeling because it's true.

Randy has frozen in his tracks with a look of confusion on his face. I brush past him barking orders as I go. "Get the oxygen tank, take vitals, set up an IV with D5W." The orders come faster than they can possibly be carried out, but I don't want him hesitating. I don't want him thinking about what's going on. There's no time and he's not ready for that yet.

He's at her side groping frantically for an elusive pulse. "Forget it," I tell him. "Get the monitor."

"But she must have a pulse, she's still conscious," he says.

One look lets him know discreetly but definitively that he is to follow my instructions to the letter without hesitation. THIS is the call that requires the strong leadership approach.

"Start CPR – she's out." Our hands are slipping and sliding on her cool clammy skin as we compress her sternum.

An hour later we're in the emergency room writing the report, cleaning equipment, re-stocking the ambulance and getting ready for the next call. Physically and emotionally we're exhausted. Our patient is dead.

"Why didn't the doctor work on her longer?" Randy asks. I survey the ambulance. Empty syringes are strewn everywhere. Drops of blood have dried on the floor. Empty packages from airways and EKG electrodes rest on the seat and the suction unit is filled with emesis. The oxygen cylinders need refilling. What more could have been done?

We see the daughter of the deceased as we leave. Her tear-stained face tells us she's already been told.

"I'm sorry," I stammer. "I wish we could have done more." It seems so inadequate, but what can I say? What can she say? There are no words.

The station house is quiet. I haven't seen Randy for a while and go in search for him. The dim light of the single lamp in the bedroom betrays the tears in his eyes. He rubs his eyes pretending to yawn. He is visibly shaken.

There are times when you need to be alone and there are times when you need to talk. Which time is this? Does this kid have what it takes to survive in this business?

My instincts tell me to leave him alone. We'll talk later. I hope I'm right.

Where are the glory calls?

2.   7,000 And Counting

There is no way to know for sure. I stopped counting after the first month of a career that has thus far spanned 14 years, but my best estimate is that I have answered those calls for help about 7,000 times.

7,000 times is a lot of times to do anything. Common sense would seem to dictate that after doing something 7,000 times, it becomes routine. In this case, common sense would be wrong.

There is nothing routine about any ambulance call. From the basic life support non-emergency transfer to the advanced life support cardiac arrest, every call is different.

Every patient is different, every partner is different, and every set of circumstances is different. Every run has the potential to make you look like a hero or a fool, and in reality you are neither. There is nothing routine about a career in EMS (emergency medical services). It is a constant challenge; one which never lets you get too comfortable with what you're doing. As soon as you get something figured out, the rules change. That's the nature of the beast.

There is nothing routine about the men and women who choose to be emergency medical technicians.

The glory-seekers disappear the first time a patient vomits on them.

The would-be doctors don't like crawling under overturned cars and getting soaked with gasoline.

The weak-hearted have trouble dealing with the patient who has been found dead after a few days.

Those with too big a heart shudder at the thought of having to triage a mass casualty disaster – letting some victims die to attend to those with a better chance of survival.

I don't like being vomited on or being soaked with gasoline. I'm not particularly fond of the warning my nose delivers when I'm about to discover a decomposed corpse. I, too, shudder at the thought of having to decide to let some people die because I don't have the resources to deal with everyone. But I put myself in a position where I might need to do these things at anytime, anyway.

This brings me to my next point. <u>We must all be crazy!</u>

After 14 years, I'm thoroughly convinced of that.

3. Then, Now, When?

The call came in to our station at about 6:00 p.m. on Thanksgiving Day. The caller thought her mother was having a heart attack.

The year was 1960.

We rushed to the scene and found a 62 year-old female with crushing substernal chest pain radiating to her left arm. She was diaphoretic and in severe distress.

I worked for a funeral home.

We put her in the back of the funeral home ambulance and raced like crazy to the hospital; running a few cars off the road as we went.

Somewhere between her home and the hospital she died. The ER doctor made the pronouncement of death.

The call came in to our station at about 6:00 pm on Thanksgiving Day. The caller thought her mother was having a heart attack.

The year was 1970.

We rushed to the scene and found a 62 year-old female with crushing substernal chest pain radiating to her left arm. She was diaphoretic and in severe distress.

I was an EMT for a volunteer ambulance service trained in basic life support.

I gave her 10 liters/minute oxygen with a face mask, recorded her vitals, put her in the back of the ambulance, and raced like crazy to the hospital; running a few cars off the road as we went.

Somewhere between her house and the hospital she died. We started CPR (cardiopulmonary resuscitation).

The ER doctor successfully resuscitated her, but she had suffered a major heart attack. She went home a month later and lived one more year as a cardiac cripple.

The call came in to our station at about 6:00 pm on Thanksgiving Day. The caller thought her mother was having a heart attack.

The year was 1980.

We rushed to the scene and found a 62 year-old female with crushing substernal chest pain radiating to her left arm. She was diaphoretic and in severe distress.

I was a paramedic for a professional ambulance service trained in advanced life support.

I gave her 10 liters/minute oxygen with a face mask and recorded her vitals. I hooked up the EKG monitor to show the heart's rhythm and started an IV. I gave four milligrams of morphine through the IV to ease the pain, reduce the work load of the heart, and put my patient at ease during transport – all of which would help to limit the size of the heart attack. I put her in the back of the ambulance and started driving quietly to the hospital to keep my patient calm.

Somewhere between her house and the hospital she developed an irregular heartbeat. I picked the appropriate anti-arrhythmic medication and gave it through the IV, thereby stabilizing the heart.

The ER doctor admitted her to the coronary care unit with a minor heart attack. A week later she went home. She enrolled in a multiphase cardiac rehabilitation program. A few months later, despite a small area of permanently damaged heart muscle, she was in better condition than she had been for the last 20 years.

The call came in to our station at about 6:00 pm on Thanksgiving Day. The caller thought her mother was having a heart attack.

12

The year was 2010.

We rushed to the scene and found a 62 year-old female with crushing substernal chest pain radiating to her left arm. She was diaphoretic and in severe distress.

I was a medical specialist, fourth grade, for the Department of Emergency Services.

I gave her 10 liter/minute oxygen. I waved my Diag-Med over her forehead, throat, chest and wrists. It gave me instantaneous readouts of her pulse, blood pressure, cardiac output, respiratory status, blood gases, electrolytes, cardiac enzymes, and 15 lead EKG.

I was surprised to see my patient was indeed having a heart attack. Preventative medicine had almost wiped out heart disease. I hadn't treated a heart attack patient for about two years.

I punched in my access number and Rescue Roy, my metallic partner, handed me the gun of polyvalent cardiac-tagged streptokinase. The gun shot the exact dose in a thousand microscopic high pressure streams right through my patient's skin.

I didn't use this stuff much anymore. Multi-tope iodine concentrate was the frequent drug these days – for radiation sickness.

The drug did its job; cleaning out the coronary arteries and reversing the heart attack. It also included a small dose of anti-arrhythmic agent to protect against cardio-lectric vulnerability during the next few high risk hours.

I advised my patient to plug into her Meda-Home computer program and to run a thorough profile to determine the cause of her problem. That way she could be assured it wouldn't happen again.

Then I left with Rescue-Roy in my jet-air scooter.

Actually, calls one and two were before I became involved in ambulance service, although I have worked for level 2 services. (Some of the rookies I work with claim I've been around since the days of bloodletting.) Call #3 is based on an actual call as are most of the others in this book. Call #4 is a vision of the future through the slightly twisted mind of a medic.

They show the differences and potential that exists all within a relatively short time span. Unfortunately, calls 1, 2, and 3 also show the differences that exist today.

Most of the major cities have the capabilities demonstrated in call #3.

Very few areas are still served by the level of care shown in call #1.

A shocking number of areas, many highly populated, still have only the basic life support found in call #2.

The main excuse used is cost. Higher quality care does cost money.

If you could upgrade the level of your ambulance service from basic to advanced life support for $10-$15/year per household, would it be worth it to you? How much is your life worth to you? What about your family's lives?

Isn't it time to have a serious talk with your politicians?

It's difficult to plan for level 4 when you're still stuck in levels 1 and 2.

4. Day One

I arrived at the station at approximately 6:15 PM for my 7:00 PM shift. My uniform was cleaned and pressed. The name pin on my pocket flap proclaimed to the world that I was "Walter Mueller, Ambulance Technician" and the patch on my shoulder told them I worked for the Volunteer Ambulance Corp.

I had carefully placed my American Red Cross Advanced First Aid Card and my American Heart Association CPR Card in my wallet so I could provide instant proof of my achievements to anyone who might doubt my credentials.

The Emergency Childbirth Course was the only thing I hadn't completed yet. If we were called on to deliver a baby, one of the other crew members would have to handle it. I would handle anything else.

Anything else???

From nowhere, butterflies suddenly appeared in my stomach and my palms grew sweaty.

Anything else??????

I had felt a warm glow of pride when I paraded to the station in my uniform for the world to see. I was here to save the world.

But when the medic I relieved went home early because I had foolishly reported before my appointed time, the warm glow quickly gave way to a sudden chill. Despite the presence of my fellow crew members, I felt very lonely.

No matter how ingeniously someone tried to hurt himself or others, I was expected to do something about it. No matter what happened, I had to handle it. There was no one I could call for help – I was the one being called to help.

What would I do if the Soviet Union picked this moment to drop the bomb on my town? What the hell was I doing here?

In comparison, Randy Whitman would look like a seasoned pro when he became a rookie years later. He would show nervousness and confusion. I was showing panic and terror.

My thirty hours of hard study in first aid and CPR seemed like nothing now. I wasn't sure I would live long enough to ever learn what I needed to know.

I probably would have left right then and never returned, except the medic I relieved was already gone. I was stuck.

Fate was kind and delivered a string of calls before I could worry myself into a heart attack.

Mrs. Winston was a jolly old lady who had celebrated her 100th birthday a few days earlier. She had fallen in her apartment and sustained a laceration to her head. As with all scalp lacerations it had bled profusely and looked horrible. Despite its appearance, however, it was a relatively minor injury.

It was readily controlled with a pressure dressing applied with a trembling hand. (I guess the stuff they teach in class really does work.)

Mrs. Winston had an unshakable demeanor – the type which can only be acquired through years of experience and wisdom.

"You boys can't carry me downstairs. I'll walk," she told us. "You'll break your backs trying to carry and old tub of lard like me."

Of course, we couldn't let her walk and she finally acquiesced.

"Sophie, stop bawling like a baby," she admonished her daughter. "You've seen blood before, there's no need to carry on so."

Truthfully, I was more concerned with the possibility of Sophie, (who was in her seventies) having a heart attack than I was about Mrs. Winston's head injury.

The call went very well and so did the next six that followed. By the end of the shift my outlook had brightened considerably.

The butterflies had returned once while enroute to an attempted suicide, but they quickly abated when we got there. Phil was an old friend to the rest of my crew who had picked him up too many times to remember. He had skillfully sliced his leg with a razor blade giving us all an anatomy lesson on the internal structure of the leg with the neat 2 inch square window he created. The call was more like a reunion between old friends than a medical emergency.

7:00 AM rolled around and it was time to leave. No one could have asked for better care than I had delivered.

I proudly paraded home in my slightly wrinkled uniform. I could handle anything.

Rookies sure are dumb.

5. Magic

The earliest days of my career were spent under the watchful eye of my first shift captain, Fernando.

Fernando was an experienced medic who worked professionally for the Peterson ambulance service as well as volunteering his time with us. He was the type of guy who doesn't just provide emergency service, he lives it every second of the day and every day of his life.

He filled in many of the gaps that were left by my initial training. While other crews watched TV or played pool between calls, Fernando was busy giving me lessons or holding practice sessions. He always encouraged me to enroll in the emergency medical technician courses.

It didn't take long for me to develop a great deal of respect for Fernando. Calls always went smoother and I felt a lot more comfortable when he was around.

Despite these qualities, Fernando was the butt of some good-natured joking around the station. Anyone who is that intense is bound to be perceived as fanatical by some and Fernando was no exception. Truthfully, he probably did go beyond reasonable limits in some things. This was probably most true of his report writing.

Back in those days ambulance run reports were not nearly the quality they are today. Even by today's standards, however, Fernando's reports were a bit excessive.

I was sitting around shooting the bull one day with a couple of guys from another shift when one of them pulled out one of Fernando's run reports and started reading it. We all chuckled when we discovered he had documented how he had carried the patient down exactly 14 stairs.

It all started as good-natured fun but as it progressed it started to change into a vicious character assassination.

As the mood of the conversation changed I found myself feeling very uncomfortable. A glance around the room told me I was not alone.

Tony was sitting in a corner of the room. Tony was a long standing member of the fire department and the president of our ambulance corps. He was known more for his quick-thinking logic, hard work and dedication than for his medical knowledge. He was also known as an emotional man who never had any trouble finding a way to express himself.

Miscommunication was never a problem with Tony. When he was speaking everyone in the building knew exactly what he was saying. Tony didn't know any official sign language, but anyone could understand the exact meaning of the Italian sign language he used.

As I watched him now, I saw his mood darkening in response to the change in the conversation. It was obvious to anyone who saw him that Tony was about to express himself again. The only question was how. I braced myself.

When it came I was surprised at how mild and self-controlled it was – by Tony's standards.

"You fucking bastards can criticize Fernando all day long but not one of you mother-fuckers is half the medic he is," Tony started out in a booming voice. "I responded to a call in a dance club and found Fernando there in a tuxedo with his band. He was doing CPR on some poor bastard who was in cardiac arrest. He had blood and vomit all over his face and his tuxedo but he never missed a fucking compression or ventilation. I've never seen any of you assholes do that. When I have my big one, he's the guy I want taking care of me."

With that he stomped out of the room before he might get upset and lose control.

The mood in the room changed once again. This time the scene reminded me of little of puppy dogs with their tails between their legs.

I left for a much needed breath of fresh air.

I was fortunate enough to be working with Fernando the first time I had a patient in cardiac arrest.

She was a 78-year-old, 225 lb. woman who was found in the upstairs bathroom by her daughter. No one knew how long she had been there. She had a long history of heart disease, hypertension, and diabetes.

When we got to her she was blue throughout the head, neck and into the chest. Her mouth was filled with vomitus and her pupils were fixed and dilated.

We cleared her airway, did CPR for a few minutes, and rushed her down the stairs. At the bottom of the stairs we resumed CPR while taking her out to the ambulance.

While enroute to the hospital she regained a spontaneous pulse. We continued to ventilate her.

By the time we got to the hospital she was moaning and starting to come around.

Despite this the ER doctor started doing chest compressions on her. I didn't understand why buy I figured it was just because I was inexperienced. Now, 14 years later, I still don't understand why.

What surprised me even more was that the doctor was doing the compressions on her left breast instead of on her breastbone as we had been taught. We were told in class that incorrect hand position decreases the effectiveness of the compressions while increasing the risk of internal injuries. This principle is still stressed in CPR classes. I still don't understand.

Anyway, despite the terrible condition in which we initially found her and despite the "care" she received in the hospital, our patient survived and ended up going home.

Of course I was happy to hear the good news; but I had expected it all along. Being a rookie, I didn't realize how small her chances were under those circumstances.

Now, after about 100 cardiac arrest patients, she is the only un-witnessed cardiac arrest patient not receiving CPR on my arrival who survived. I can't help wondering if Fernando might have been blessed with a special magical touch.

6.   Evicted

My ears perked up when I first heard the faint siren off in the distance. After a few seconds of intent listening I knew it was getting closer.

Was it police, fire or ambulance? Suddenly the air horn blared and I knew it was the fire department. In a short while I could feel the house trembling beneath my feet as a pumper raced down my street.

Instead of fading gradually, the siren stopped abruptly. They were nearby. It was no big deal yet. Over half of the 1500 annual fire alarms in our city were false alarms.

When there was a working fire, however, it was always a big deal. You see, our city has an estimated actual population of about 70,000 people crammed into about 1-1/12 square miles. It is a city of old, dilapidated houses jammed to standing room only. The buildings stand side by side with little or no space in between. Any fire that isn't rapidly extinguished spreads quickly from one fire trap to the next with a horrendous potential for loss of life.

Our city would have burned to the ground years ago if they had anything less than the best fire department. There are four firehouses in this small city with a total force of over 120 paid firemen. In addition, the mutual aid agreements with neighboring towns are exercised regularly. They are quick and they are good. In the five years I worked on the ambulance corps, they never lost a civilian life – an amazing feat considering the circumstances.

I remember listening to their sirens as a kid and running out to find the excitement. In some towns a multiple alarm fire doesn't even guarantee the sight of flames. This was not the case here. The numerous scenes I witnessed were filled with towering flames, blackened skies, scurrying firemen, and a strong odor of smoke.

Now I was listening for the sirens again, but for a different reason. In my fourth month of duty on the ambulance corps, I had not yet been to a major fire scene. There had been several, but not while I was around.

In another minute I heard a second siren approaching. This was it! A second alarm had been turned in. It was a major working fire.

I ran outside, looked for the telltale plume of smoke and ran toward it. Even though I was off duty, it would be my chance to experience a working fire as a medic. I was there within three minutes of the time I heard the first siren stop. The ambulance was already there with a patient inside.

A 25-year-old woman had sustained first and second degree burns to her back before being rescued by the fire department. Working on her inside the ambulance were Hector (who I had just met briefly since we didn't work on the same shift) and his wife, Joannie (who I had seen on station once but not been introduced to yet).

26

This was a great opportunity to learn how to care for burns first-hand, but as I climbed in the rear door of the ambulance, Joannie squared off in front of me blocking my path.

"You'll have to wait outside," she informed me somewhat brusquely.

"Okay," I said falling backward out of the ambulance. I had seen five people crowd into the back of an ambulance to work on a patient. There was no doubt that was too many. There wasn't even room to move. This time, though, only Hector and Joannie were back there. Well, maybe they liked lots of elbow room.

I figured I could learn just as easily by watching through the tiny windows in the rear door of the ambulance. I climbed on the rear bumper-step for a better view. The chassis gave way under my weight alerting the ever vigilant Joannie to my current whereabouts.

She charged the rear door, flinging it outward and once again toppling me backward off the ambulance.

"<u>Please</u> stay away from the ambulance," she insisted. "I'll let you know when you can come in."

Well, maybe I was a rookie, but even so she had no right to treat a fellow squad member that way. I climbed back up determined to watch whether Joannie wanted me to or not.

This time I was prepared and sidestepped the door when she threw it open. The torrent of verbal abuse spewing from her mouth, however, caught me completely off guard.

"You disgusting creep," she yelled at me. "What are you, some kind of pervert hoping for a free show? Get away from here right now before I have the cops arrest you."

I fell backward off the ambulance once again. (I fell backward off the ambulance more times in those few minutes than I have in the subsequent 14 years of my career.)

I was completely dumbfounded. Nothing like this had ever happened to me before. As the newest rookie I had been the target of numerous pranks and put-downs but never to this extent and never in the presence of a patient.

For a few minutes I just stood around wondering what to do next. Finally I got up the nerve to peer inside one more time (carefully avoiding stepping on the bumper).

Inside I saw Hector talking to Joannie. Joannie was just sitting there with her mouth hanging open. Then she came to the door. (I hurriedly jumped back ten feet in a single bound when I saw her coming.) She timidly told me I could come in now.

Inside she smiled a weak grin and explained that she hadn't recognized me and thought that I was a friend of the patient. When the patient denied knowing me she assumed I was just a bystander.

We became good friends despite our rocky beginning and she never threw me out of an ambulance again.

Neither has anyone else.

7. My Home Town

I never really knew the kinds of things that went on in my home town until I started working ambulance there. When I did, I was shocked by some of the things I saw.

I never thought I lived a sheltered life but I had no idea of the number of assaults, child abuse, arson, rapes, neglect of the young and elderly, etc. that was going on in this small but densely-populated town in a busy metropolitan area.

We pulled up outside the bar in our ambulance. The police were already there. The call had come in to us as a shooting inside the bar.

As I jumped out I was surprised to see the bar dark and closed. It was only 1:00 AM on a Saturday night. The bars here stayed open until 3:00 AM.

Our patient was lying in a pool of blood outside. He was dead.

The caller must have been mistaken, I figured.

Not so.

On the way back to the station I was informed that this was the usual procedure. Whenever someone was shot or stabbed in a barroom fight, the bar would empty out. The bartender would then drag the body out to the street, lock up the place and go home. One of the patrons would invariably experience pangs of guilt after getting home and make an anonymous phone call to us. This was the routine way of doing things in this neighborhood.

So several years and a few more of these calls later I thought I knew what to expect as I responded to a call of a "Man down in a bar".

Not so.

This patient had a relatively minor scalp laceration. He had been dragged out to the street as was customary but I couldn't find anything severe enough to have caused his death.

Several days later I learned the coroner's report had shown the cause of death to be a heart attack.

Apparently he had suffered his heart attack while in the bar. He must have fallen unconscious to the floor, striking his head on the corner of the bar as he fell.

No one in the bar knew for sure what happened. They just knew there was a dead man in the bar with a head wound. Fearing the worst, they dragged him out to the street, locked the place up, went home, and made the obligatory anonymous phone call.

I'm glad I don't live there anymore.

8. Hector

The short guy with the gimpy walk, short black hair and a black moustache was walking toward me grinning broadly as always.

If you gave him only a superficial glance and you were the type of person out to cause trouble, you might consider him an easy mark.

If you were this type of person and made this error, you would pay dearly for your mistake with a lesson you would never forget.

A closer examination would reveal muscles rippling all over his body. They were not the massive show off muscles developed by body builders. These were functional muscles meant for hard physical labor. Solid.

A glance at his eyes revealed a level of intelligence that transcended his apparently carefree countenance.

Every little movement he made gave the impression that it was the best movement he could possibly make at that time, accomplished with both flair and precision. I don't know if this was due to his martial arts expertise, or if that expertise came about because of the fluidity and efficiency of his movements.

This is Hector.

"Hey Walt, I heard you want to be in my EMT course," he said. "Have you gotten hold of an application yet?"

Some people are born with a gift. They have a particular talent for something and can excel at it effortlessly.

Others have a burning compulsion to work at some particular task until it is perfected. Nothing stands in their way and they work tirelessly day and night to achieve an unparalleled level of excellence.

About once in a lifetime, I suppose, you find an individual who combines both of these qualities. Someone who could be the best without even trying but who isn't satisfied with merely being the best.

The only acceptable level of achievement for these people is the next highest one regardless of the level they're at.

This is Hector.

In addition to his volunteer work, Hector worked full time for a neighboring city's paid professional ambulance service. Working in that much larger city made our volunteer work look like a child's playground. Hector had the opportunity to hone his considerable martial arts skills at least weekly there.

Besides his ambulance work, Hector was also the county coordinator for the Emergency Medical Technician (EMT) course. The fact that he is as good a teacher as he is a field medic has aided my own career immeasurably, as well as the careers of many others, I'm sure.

Hector challenged, prodded, and taught me throughout that EMT course with the result that I passed with flying colors and was recommended for instructor training.

If you want to learn something, study it. If you want to absorb it, teach it.

I started working with one of the most elite groups of instructors I have ever known.

Hector's efforts as coordinator were assisted admirably by his wife, Joannie. (Yes, this is the same Joannie who kept tossing me out of the ambulance.) Joannie's own level of skill and dedication was admirable and she took a back seat to no one.

Beyond Hector and Joannie was a central core of instructors composed of Charlie and Pat and Joe, all volunteers in their respective towns.

This group was assisted by myself and several other new graduates.

Our task was formidable.

Take a class of about 100 completely untrained and inexperienced people. Toss out the jokers, the insincere and those looking for a few easy credits from a simple first aid course. This leaves about 50 students.

34

Of these 50, weed out the ones who are physically, mentally or emotionally incapable of being good field medics.

This leaves about 35.

In a three month period, these 35 people would be transformed into medics, ready to face the rigors of a career in EMS.

At the end of each course, we always gave our 35 graduates this warning: "You now have barely enough training to go out and start learning on your own."

On an average I suppose about four or five people from each course lasted longer than three years in the field.

It wasn't exactly a high percentage; but it was the highest in the state. Those that did survive are invaluable assets to their communities.

From Hector I learned to observe and learn from everyone. Even a poor medic might have some little trick that might make things easier. Sometimes I learned about pitfalls to avoid.

The end result is that my skills and knowledge are a compilation of the skills and knowledge of hundreds of medics I have worked with.

The new rookies can learn from those hundreds of medics through me and add their own skills and experience to become better than I am.

It's a grand pyramid scheme in which everyone wins.

Beyond improving my own knowledge and teaching skills, what else did I learn from the rest of these elite instructors I worked with?

"Bull's eye," yelled Pat with a big smile on his face.

"No way," shouted Charlie, running to the dart board. "See, here's the hole. It's not even close."

Pat was furious. "That's not the hole you crazy half-blind bastard. There's the hole, right in the center of the bull's eye."

"Don't give me any of your crap," Charlie yelled pushing Pat.

"You want to make something of it?"

"What are you going to do about it?"

Throughout it all Joe sat in a corner reciting colorful limericks and laughing raucously after each one.

People started to leave. The bartender rolled his eyes, hung his head in his hands, and resigned himself to another slow night at the hands of his select clientele, the county vocational school's EMT instructors.

This was not a pansy bar. Customers didn't leave here just because of an argument. The bartender would calmly call for the police and then continue to serve drinks during any fist fights here.

Charlie and Pat's playful argument sounded real enough to anyone who didn't know them well. Even so, this was not why people were leaving.

Every Thursday night after teaching EMT class Hector, Joannie, Charlie, Pat, Joe and I came here for a few drinks. We soon realized we never saw the same customers twice. Once they realized we were coming in on Thursdays, they avoided the place leaving us with a new crowd to break in.

We had been closely scrutinized when we entered like always. People began to fidget nervously when Charlie and Pat went to the dart board.

You see, there were no darts. The bartender had taken them away months ago when Charlie and Pat started playing catch with them.

A silence had fallen over the bar as Charlie and Pat played a few rounds, carefully keeping track of the score and paying each other off for bets won.

The argument over the imaginary dart game, however, was too much even for the most stoic of barroom crowds and they all fled to find a saner corner of the world.

From these people, the most dedicated and experienced EMS professionals I have ever known, I learned to be crazy.

I learned to match my dedication to EMS with an equal dedication to relaxation and good times.

This lesson has probably done more to prolong my career than any other.

9. Ambulance People

Unfortunately not everyone who works on an ambulance is there because of a burning desire to help people. Some people are just there for the excitement, the image, or the glory whether real or imagined.

These people are easy to pick out. They are the ones with more medals, badges, patches, trim, and gold braid on their uniforms than a five star general in full dress uniform. They have pagers and radios protruding from every pocket all of which are blaring at the same time in an incomprehensible cacophony of static.

There are other telltale signs, too. These people are never seen in training sessions. They have no idea where the equipment is stored or even what it is used for. They have only one seat they will use in the ambulance – the driver's seat. From this position they can fondle the switches for the lights and siren they love so dearly.

If you're looking for one of these people you better look quickly. They don't last very long.

Harry was one of those people. As a matter of fact, he fit the description perfectly. His self-esteem was measured by how many radio antennas he had on his car.

Harry's exaggerated attempts to impress the public with his importance led to his own public humiliation and downfall.

I was sitting in a diner eating breakfast with Harry. We were both off duty and had just met accidentally. Even Harry's civilian clothes were covered with official looking patches and he had his ever-present hand-held scanner sitting on the table. It was the type of scanner with which you could pick up four different frequencies at once. It was only used for listening, however. You couldn't transmit with it.

Harry was desperately trying to impress our waitress. I could see the wheels turning in his head and I knew something bizarre was about to happen.

Finally, a plan formulated in his mind.

He jumped up from the table raising his scanner to his face as he did so.

"This is the chief," he yelled at the top of his lungs. "I'm responding from the other side of town. I'll be there in two minutes. I'll save that patient's life."

Then he turned to me. "Come on Mueller, they need help and I might be able to use your assistance."

With that he ran outside leaving me laughing hysterically at the table.

Harry's car was parked right in front of the diner in full view of everyone. We could all see Harry fumbling desperately looking for his keys – the keys which were sitting on the table in front of me.

By the time he came back inside to retrieve his keys, everyone in the diner was doubled over with laughter.

"What's so funny?" he demanded gruffly.

He growled at me, snatched the keys off the table and ran outside again.

The laughter died down just enough to hear whrr, whrr, whrr. Harry couldn't get the car started.

A second wave of laughter swept the diner as I found myself gasping for air.

Harry stepped out of the car, slammed the door shut and walked to the bus stop.

The diner finally quieted down and everyone returned to their breakfast in a much more jovial mood than they started in.

The story of Harry's little escapade spread like wildfire through the ambulance service.

I suppose it was mean of me to let the story out in the first place. However, it was nicer than locking him in a closet all day, embarrassing him in front of nurses, or kicking him out of the ambulance in some rough neighborhood.

These were all techniques which had been used on other ambulance people who didn't belong. They are very effective techniques for getting rid of unwanted ambulance people.

You may have noticed I never refer to Harry as a medic. He wasn't a medic. He was an ambulance person. He was until the diner incident anyway.

Some people don't belong on ambulance crews. Many of them are good and sincere people who for one reason or another cannot or choose not to continue in the EMS field. These people are fine. They are reasonable people who try something they think would fit them. When they realize it does not, they leave.

The Harry-type person, however, never leaves willingly. He is so consumed with his image that he is blind to the threat he poses to his patients and fellow crew members.

The majority of medics are hardworking dedicated people who will do almost anything to help a patient. They back up their partners even under risk of physical harm. These things are simply assumed to be the medic's duty.

The average medic is far more substance than appearance. You might not be impressed if you meet one on the street, but you will be when you have your heart attack.

True medics cannot and will not tolerate Harry. They will do whatever is necessary to make Harry's career as short as possible.

It's a good thing for you they do.

10. Every Size, Shape, and Color

What kind of person becomes a medic?

Black people do. So do white people, yellow people, and probably green and purple people too.

Many Christians become medics. Many Jews become medics. Buddhists, atheists, Muslims and agnostics all become medics.

Medics are Democrats, Republicans, and Independents.

They are upper class, lower class, and middle class.

Size and sex used to be discriminating factors for medics. A medic's job does not consist of continuous hard labor. It does, however, involve short but unpredictable periods of intense physical exertion as well as an occasional risk of personal danger.

It may have never been a written policy, but it was always assumed that a large guy could deal with these problems better than a small guy and any guy could deal with them better than any girl.

I remember being challenged to a wrestling match. I am 6' 3" and weigh 200 lbs... I was the underdog.

My friend, crew member, and opponent was nearly as tall and outweighed me by 40 pounds. Size alone doesn't impress me. Frank impressed me. I had seen him accomplish some amazing feats of strength in the time we had worked together.

However, Frank was slow. I knew speed and quickness were on my side so I accepted the challenge.

The match lasted a full fifteen seconds. It should probably be in the Guinness Book of World Records.

Frank picked me up and started spinning me in the air over his head. I immediately realized there were only three possible outcomes. I could wait for Frank to slam-dunk me to finish me off. I could wait for Frank to get tired and drop me. I could concede the match. Somehow, I didn't find the first two possibilities appealing.

So much for speed and quickness.

I must admit I enjoyed being the smallest guy on my crew. There were times when it was a definite advantage. I could hide behind those guys and no one would even know I was there.

Eventually, however, I learned size and sex are mostly a psychological advantage. Sometimes you can get out of a tough spot simply by looking big without ever having to prove yourself. When you do have to prove yourself, however, size has no advantage and neither does sex.

Our 250 pound patient was lying on the floor, disabled by a stroke. He was conscious and his vitals were stable. I had reassured his wife that he was cognizant of what was happening by having him squeeze her hand on command; he couldn't talk.

The problem we faced was not a medical one. We were eight floors high in a building with a broken elevator. (Ambulance Rule #1 is that whenever you're on the fourth floor or higher, the elevator is either broken or too small to use.)

I was working for Central Ambulance, a private non-emergency transfer service, and there was no one I could call for assistance.

Kevin, my partner, was ready to go. We had worked together often and I was always amazed at the way his 5'4" 120 pound body would respond to any challenge. His baby face always had a smile on it and he would never win a John Wayne lookalike contest, but he was tough. He was as tough as they come. Kevin was 100% heart and desire. He never questioned whether or not he could do a job; he simply went ahead and did it.

Eight flights of stairs with a 250 pound patient, however, is a lot to ask of anyone. At least our patient was stable. There was no rush and we could stop and rest on every landing if Kevin needed to.

After the sixth flight, I looked at Kevin with a red face, bulging eyes, sore and trembling muscles, and begged him to stop for a rest.

"Sure," Kevin said, smiling like always.

"He's just lucky there's no kryptonite around," I thought.

I have seen small men and women who could out-lift, out-carry, and out-fight many men twice their size.

One reason they can do this is because they don't try to muscle their way through everything. They use their head and employ good technique. Thus, you see more monster-sized medics suffering with back problems than normal sized ones. Good technique can go a long way toward avoiding serious problems, but it isn't the answer to every situation.

One of the hospitals I worked with had their chief physical therapist give us an in-service one day on the proper way to lift and move patients. He demonstrated to us all the proper techniques for lifting a patient out of bed, transferring a patient from one cot to another, and even for lifting a patient from the ground. When he finished he asked us if we had any questions.

"What's the proper technique for carrying a patient down a flight of stairs?" we inquired.

A perplexed look came over his face. "You should never do that," he told us.

We just smiled.

Big medics tend to believe they can handle anything simply because they are big. Small medics are more prone to keeping themselves in good shape.

You also need good concentration. Losing concentration, even for a second, can hurt.

I lost my concentration once while carrying a patient down a single flight of stairs. My knee still reminds me of it occasionally. The twinge of pain I get isn't nearly as bad as the memory it invokes of the excruciating pain I felt when it happened.

Good technique, staying in shape, good concentration, and a healthy dose of luck are the key ingredients to surviving the physical aspects of this business. Large size really doesn't enter the picture.

Unfortunately, women and small men are often discriminated against. They are often required to prove themselves before being hired. This isn't a bad idea. However, it should be required of everyone. I've seen female applicants pass physical fitness tests that half the guys on the service would flunk.

My doubts about working with small people were erased early in my career when Sue and I carried a 350 pound patient down two flights of stairs. I often wish my male partners had her ability.

About the only discriminating factor left for medics is age. Most medics tend to be young. The majority leaves the field before turning 30 and only a handful make it to 40.

The physical requirements of the job are one reason for this. A far bigger reason is the politics of the job.

Medic salaries are not real good in most places. As a matter of fact, many services are still completely volunteer.

Volunteers are a mixed blessing. There is no doubt they perform a much-needed service while saving their community a lot of money.

There is also no doubt that the same volunteers, given full time jobs, could develop greater skills and serve their community much better as professionals.

The very existence of volunteers, however, makes it easier for short-sighted politicians to rationalize not having a professional service.

Is it really so impossible to raise the money for a paid ambulance service? How much money do you spend every month for cable TV even though free TV is readily available to you? For less money than that you could change your ambulance service from volunteer to professional. Which is more important to you?

The very politicians who are supposed to run many ambulance services are often directly responsible for shortening the careers of medics. Politics enters the ambulance decision making process far too often and many medics have been unjustly fired or harassed and discouraged into quitting.

Why should politicians have near total control over an ambulance service? Granted there are often public funds involved and some political oversight is warranted.

However, medical decisions and emergency service experience are vital components of the system and should receive at least equal representation. Yet many ambulance services are ruled almost entirely by a purely political board.

I worked as a volunteer in my home town for five years only to have the mayor and several of his cohorts thrown in jail for corruption. I thought I was helping the community by saving them money, but the community wasn't getting the money I saved. They would have been better off spending it on a professional ambulance service (which they still don't have).

Volunteers have all the same qualities as paid medics do, but they could be much more effective as better-trained full time professionals.

If a medic survives the possibility of outright political firing, does not allow himself to be discouraged by political ignorance and interference, can tolerate the low pay and worse benefits, and can keep his mental and physical capacities sharp, he can look forward to a long career in EMS.

If not, the community will bear both the financial and medical costs of maintaining a work force in a field with one of the highest turnover rates around.

11. The Sixth Sense

We're supposed to be the eyes, ears and hands of the physician out in the streets. That's what they tell us. There's no denying that all five of the senses play an important role in emergency medical service; but they're not the most important.

The sixth sense has never been clearly defined in any anatomy text. People argue over its existence as if there was really doubt. If you doubt the existence of the sixth sense, just ask any seasoned EMT. He will not only confirm its existence for you; he will tell you what it is.

The sixth sense is your gut. When things are looking great but butterflies inexplicably appear in your gut, something is wrong. Some subtle change for the worse is occurring that your other five senses can't discern yet, but your gut knows. When your gut feels like it just dropped 1,000 feet in one second – Watch Out!!! A 747 is probably falling from the skies and is going to land right on top of your ambulance.

A good gut is the best tool an EMT has. Ignoring your gut instincts can be fatal.

The call sounded innocent enough when it came in. A woman was having a heart attack. Ernie, Joannie and I rushed in to help.

We found a heavy set woman clutching her chest in a back corner of a small crowded basement apartment. There were ten or twelve people there who we assumed to be family. Everyone there, including our patient, was speaking Spanish. We did not.

Ernie went out for the cot while Joannie and I continued our examination of the patient. The butterflies were in my stomach. I didn't know why and I was too busy tending to my patient to bother to find out.

Suddenly the conversation in the room became noticeably louder. The next moment fists were flying, feet were kicking, people were screaming, and we found ourselves in the middle of a riot.

Ernie observed all this from outside and called in for police assistance. He kind of lost his cool on the radio, but when you think about it, that's the best way to let the police know that you want them here Right Now!

Joannie (who was pregnant at the time) and I were still in the corner with our patient. We were uninvolved so far, but we couldn't get out.

A seventeen-year-old kid was going at it pretty good with an older guy who was next to me. The kid ran over to the wall to get something and when I saw what it was, my gut dropped 1,000 feet. There was a machete hanging on the wall! (Some people are great interior decorators.)

There is a certain amount of danger in being an EMT. I had faced it before. It is not as much as firemen who make a career out of rushing into burning buildings. It is not as much as policemen who get called into riots by people like me who should have known better than to be in there in the first place. But the danger is there, and any rookie cop could tell you that domestic quarrels present the most potential for danger.

I had faced knives before and on very rare occasions even a gun. I would be lying if I told you I wasn't scared to death, but I had always managed to walk away unscathed.

Machetes, however, were new to me and I was developing an intense dislike for them.

The kid rushed his adversary (who was still standing next to Joannie and I) swinging the machete back and forth in front of him. An ugly vision of three or four heads falling to the floor with one mighty swoop entered my mind – and one of those heads was mine.

I would have to try to kick the machete from his hand. It would require critical timing and frankly I was not at all confident that I was that good. I stepped in front of Joannie and our patient and prepared for the worst.

Just before I had to find out if I was good enough, three people tackled the kid from behind. The machete somehow disappeared, the fight continued, and we were still trapped – but my head was still on my shoulders.

54

Just when I thought we could remain uninvolved, I spotted a guy throwing a six-year-old kid against the walls in the next bedroom. Adults can beat each other up all day long if they want and I'll pick up the pieces when they're done. An adult beating a child, however, is a different story. I entered the room intent on stopping him and hoping to stay alive in the process. I knew that as a stranger, if I intervened I might inadvertently unify everyone it the apartment - against me! He saw me coming, stopped and left.

That was fine with me. I had accomplished what I intended to and the kid was safe. I was using my luck rapidly and didn't want to push it any further.

The first police unit to arrive was a two man squad car. They stood outside the doorway and called in to see if we were okay. They weren't coming in until their backup got there. (I always thought that's what the purpose of a two man car was.)

The second unit to arrive was the evening superior, Sgt. Frerror. He was better known as Frerror the Terror.

He had earned this nickname by overreacting to numerous situations. The most notorious one was when he called out the troops because he saw some people in a dark alley enter an apartment building with rifles. After surrounding the building, positioning his sharpshooters, breaking out the tear gas, and calling in reinforcements; he got on the bullhorn and demanded the fugitives' surrender.

About a dozen very nervous teenagers in their high school flag corps uniforms complete with fake rifles emerged from their party and surrendered on the spot.

Now, however, I was elated to see Frerror the Terror. A little overreaction would help balance what I felt was under reaction by the first unit.

Frerror stormed in past the first two officers with riot helmet on, hand on gun, and nightstick swinging. Bodies started flying through the air and by the time the first two cops had managed to move out of the doorway, it was all over.

The hospital determined our patient had just been hysterical over the family squabble which had apparently started prior to our arrival. Joannie decided that night to take a leave of absence till after she had her baby. I promised myself never to ignore my gut again. And we all thanked Lady Luck for blessing us with more than our share.

By the way, I don't know how you feel about other weapons, but there is no question in my mind that machetes should be banned from the face of the earth forever.

12. The Bear

"Sometimes you eat the bear and sometimes the bear eats you," Conrad was saying. It was his favorite saying and I had heard it 1,000 times.

This time he was using it to explain to a rookie why he didn't get any calls on a Saturday night – generally the busiest night of the week. As volunteers we staffed a station 24/7. It was too busy for us to respond from home. Rookies like lots of calls. Old pros like lots of sleep.

The point of his argument was that you can't depend on the odds. You never know what's going to happen when. If a doctor tells me I need surgery, I don't want to know if I have an 80% chance of surviving. I want to know if I'm going to be in the 80% that survive or in the 20% that die. After all, it's really an all or nothing proposition in the end.

Unfortunately, no one I know has a crystal ball so there is really no alternative but to play the odds in your favor.

So when the country started preparing for its bicentennial, we started preparing for the imminent disaster.

The great sailing ships were scheduled to cruise down the Hudson River in a spectacular display for all to enjoy. That was the problem, there were too many "all".

The forecasts from the experts were gloomy. The stone walls lining the cliffs would give way under the unyielding force of thousands of people straining to get a better view. Scores of people would plummet to the railroad and shipping yards 100 feet below.

The balconies of the high rises lining the cliffs would be an excellent vantage point. But with all the residents and their guests on one side of the building at one time, the entire building would topple sending thousands of people to their death.

The traffic jams would turn every street for miles into a parking lot and access to or exit from the site of this disaster would be impossible.

How do you plan for a disaster of this magnitude?

1. Contact every ambulance service in the state so on the big day you can have a staffed ambulance on every other corner and teams with field packs walking between them.
2. Arrange to have refrigerated railroad cars nearby for use as a temporary morgue.
3. Buy more trauma supplies to stuff into your ambulance than you have bought for the last five years.
4. Establish an outer perimeter of ambulances, light and heavy duty rescue squads, and fire and police personnel. When the dust clears after the great

deluge, this outer perimeter would move in to see if anything can be salvaged.

It was going to be a big day for trauma injuries and none of us relished the idea. I had two ambulances, one light and one heavy duty rescue squad under my command at one of the perimeter stations. We stood by our post nervously awaiting the call to battle.

And waiting. And waiting. And waiting.

We were under orders to restrict all unnecessary radio traffic to keep the airways clear for the voluminous emergency transmissions; but there wasn't a peep. I defied orders by asking for a radio check. The radio dispatcher was quick to acknowledge my radio check. It sounded as if he was glad to hear a voice – almost as if he was lonely.

I decided to turn over my command and investigate personally.

The streets were practically deserted. They didn't even have their usual amount of traffic. Not only hadn't anyone come, people actually avoided the area.

I guess all the gloomy forecasts were a bit too much.

I bought a hot dog from a sad looking vendor. He was surrounded by mountains of frankfurters in cases of rapidly melting ice.

We had a total of seven ambulance runs that day (we generally averaged ten calls per day). Not one of them was a trauma. As a matter of fact, only one of them was worth remembering at all. It was one of those calls you never forget. It was the type of call that fits a small but important category of satisfying and rewarding calls; the kind of call that makes you glow.

For the first time in my career I assisted in the delivery of a baby that day.

Sometimes you eat the bear and sometimes the bear eats you.

Bear meat sure tastes good.

13. Donny

Support groups perform a vital social function throughout the world. Everyone has problems, worries, doubts, and fears; and support groups are an essential factor in dealing with these adversities. In general the stronger the adversity, the stronger the support group becomes.

A career in EMS includes a lot of adversity. The risks of physical attack, career assassination, and injury combined with the strain of maintaining current and efficient skill levels lead to the formation of very strong ties between crew members. The added impact of the emotional experiences shared by a crew following some calls, forge these relationships into extremely close support groups. By necessity, ambulance support groups are often stronger than those found in other social areas.

All successful ambulance crews will develop these support groups naturally. When a crew has worked together for a while, they just assume that their partner will be there to provide all the backup needed. No discussion is needed.

Very rarely is this trust violated. When it is violated, it is lost irreparably.

It is also very rare for an outsider to become part of these groups. Even rookies have a hard time being accepted. They have to prove themselves first. Thus, someone who doesn't even work in EMS can only penetrate these groups under very rare and very special occasions.

Donny is one of these people.

Donny worked for the Department of Public Works. Donny outweighed me by about 40 pounds. As for his strength, let's just say that when I suggested that my wrestling nemesis, Frank might try a match with Donny, he looked at me like I was out of my mind. He wouldn't even consider it.

Donny only had one problem. He was mentally retarded. At least most people would consider it a problem. I'm not so sure.

He was a hard working self-sufficient man. He was intelligent, at least in terms of practical day-to-day living. He was just slow. His bright red face, balding head, and high squeaky voice made him somewhat of a comical looking figure.

Most of all, Donny had a heart as big as the universe. He was a friendly easy-going man who loved everyone on sight. Nothing short of outright violence would anger him, although I did see him saddened on numerous occasions by the taunting jeers of ignorant uncaring fools. I often thought the world would be a better place if we were all more like Donny.

Everyone's favorite story was about the time Donny was robbed. Two punk teenagers demanded his wallet pretending to have guns in their pockets. Donny gave them his extra empty wallet that he always carried in case of a robbery. Street smart.

They ran away taunting him and yelling that they didn't really have guns. They were so cocky they didn't even look behind them.

Donny was following them. He was slow but he kept following and when they stopped to see what was in the wallet, he caught them.

He grabbed each one by the back of the neck using sufficient pressure to let them know they better not try anything.

Now, however, he had a dilemma. What was he going to do with them? Just then a police car passed by on this crowded street. All city workers knew Donny including the police, but Donny was afraid the cops wouldn't notice him on the busy street so he picked both kids up by the backs of their necks and waved them in the air for the cops to see.

If that isn't enough to end a budding career in crime, nothing is.

Donny hung around the ambulance station all the time. He loved us. He thought we were great for doing the things we did. He thought we were heroes. Donny was our hero.

Whenever there was a 400 plus pound patient who had to be carried down a flight of stairs (which happened more times than my back likes to remember), Donny always popped up as if by magic.

Whenever we needed to extricate a patient from a mangled car, Donny could tear the car apart with his bare hands better than we could with our tools.

Donny was also very good at saving lives – ours.

When I heard the address, I knew we were in trouble.

If you live near a large city you have probably seen TV news accounts of an ambulance crew waiting on the street for police backup before going in to a particular building to get a patient.

Newsmen seem to feel this is an unacceptable practice. Did you ever notice you never see pictures of the inside of those buildings on TV?

I'm sure every large city has buildings like that. If you're lucky enough to survive your first few calls there, you learn from experience not to go in again. If you do, one of those days you won't come out.

Some people are after drugs. Even services that don't carry drugs have been subjected to this. Some people see your uniform as a symbol of authority. Some people are just bored and want to add some excitement to their lives by bashing your skull in.

We were on our way to one of those buildings now. The caller said her husband had a stroke. It sounded legitimate.

I called for police backup. There were no units available.

Frank and I went inside moving rapidly. We would get our patient outside and start treatment in the ambulance. We found him on the second floor, got him on the stretcher, and were about to leave when Donny showed up.

"Hi guys. I saw the rig outside. Do you need any help?" he asked.

I carried the head end of the stretcher, Frank took the foot end, and I had Donny back up Frank going down the flight of stairs.

We were halfway down when two drugged out punks appeared at the bottom. They had waited for just the right moment, and this was it. Frank and I had our hands full with the patient and there was no place to set him down. Only Donny stood between us and them.

"Hey guys, get out of the way," Donny yelled, not yet realizing what was happening.

I called to him to back off but he wasn't listening to me. Then I heard two deadly clicks and saw the switchblades in their hands.

Donny saw them too. He understood now.

"You're trying to hurt these guys," he yelled at them, his voice shaking with anger.

Donny had his back to me but I could see the back of his neck and his balding head turning deep purple. He tensed and huge muscles appeared everywhere. I could even envision the ugly scowl that was on his face.

Our adversaries seemed a little less certain of their objective now.

When Donny started advancing on them, like a mountain advancing on two anthills, they fled.

I'm glad it turned out that way. You never know for sure how a fight is going to turn out and I sure wouldn't like seeing Donny get hurt.

If Donny had won, he could have hurt them terribly, maybe even killed them. Even under these circumstances, the kind-hearted Donny would have had trouble living with that kind of memory.

14. Dr. Bismo

EMS is a wonderful profession. Sure it can get tough out on the street, but when you return to the station it's a different world.

Your crew members are very supportive and willing to help in any way possible.

The other rescue agencies go out of their way to help you.

The fire department will jump for joy when you ask them to come out in the middle of the night to wash your patient's blood out of the street.

The police department loves coming out to save your hide when you've placed your hide where it shouldn't be.

When you need an expensive new piece of equipment to help you save someone's life the politicians will gladly find a way to finance it. They'll even offer to raise the property taxes 2⃞ per $100 assessed valuation to give you a raise because you do such a good job.

The public will gladly accept the tax raise and even offer to give more. After all, they realize they spend more money on garbage collection than on ambulance service.

The emergency room staff praises your work and thanks you profusely for delivering a stable cleaned up patient.

This may all seem pretty utopian to you and you may be starting to question my truthfulness; but stop and think about it.

Your fellow squad members know that whatever happens to you will sooner or later happen to them also. Their support will be returned in their time of need.

The police and fire departments are determined to establish good interdepartmental relations. After all, sooner or later they'll need your services too.

The public knows that by paying a few extra pennies in taxes they can get the best EMS anywhere – a bargain at any price.

The politicians know this will keep the public happy, thereby assuring their re-election.

The emergency room staff knows good cooperation and communication is essential to their patients' well-being, thus making their jobs easier and more satisfying.

You see, there's really no reason to believe things aren't exactly as I've told you.

If you believe any of this I have twenty bridges just waiting for a sharp investor like you to buy. All you have to do is drain the swamp land that's covering them first.

"I want to tell you about our last call before I leave," Robbie said, "Just in case you catch any flak over it."

This is not the ideal way to be greeted at the beginning of a new shift.

"We were called for a guy down by the cops," he continued. "One whiff of him and I figured he was drunk – but I couldn't arouse him even with the ammonia caps. Then he started vomiting blood. I figured we better get him in quick so I took him to the nearest hospital – Edgewood."

There were those damn butterflies again.

"The ER head nurse called just before you got here. She was pissed and wanted us out there to transfer the guy to the VA Hospital. I didn't think it was a good idea, so I refused. She threatened to report us to the nursing supervisor."

I looked at my watch. Robbie was right. It was rush hour. Our city with an estimated actual population of 70,000 was located just outside New York City. At that moment it had at least five times that many people traveling through it at breakneck speed on their way home from a hard day at the office. A non-emergency transfer to the VA Hospital now would tie up my only ambulance for at least two hours. I agreed with Richie's assessment. I just wanted to know where he got that "report us" bullshit from.

Edgewood Hospital was not a community or charity organization hospital like the others in our area. It was privately owned – mostly by Dr. Bismo. It was also brand new.

In their three week old history, we had already clashed on numerous occasions. It seems they only wanted rich people in their hospital. You can't recoup the expense of building a new hospital with welfare cases. I had personally reminded their staff on several occasions that failure to provide emergency care to a patient, regardless of the patient's ability to pay, was not only an affront to their moral responsibilities, but also a violation of their civil duty and licensure for which they could have their license suspended and be sued. I had reminded them of this in a friendly way, of course.

It took thirty minutes for the nursing supervisor to call me. I had expected her call much earlier than that. Maybe she figured I'd get nervous and crack if she gave me some time to worry about it. The same strategy is used to "ice" field goal kickers by the opposing team in football games.

It took her only a few minutes to realize no amount of shouting would change my mind. "I'm going to call Dr. Bismo," she threatened. "Okay," I said.

This time it was quicker. I don't remember for sure, but I don't think I even had time to sit down again before the phone was ringing.

70

"Get your ass over to my hospital and get that bum out of there," boomed an authoritative voice.

"Who's calling please?" I asked.

A burst of steam shot out of the phone receiver.

"You know damn well who this is. Get that drunk out of my hospital. Take him to the VA, take him home, dump him on the street. I don't care but get him out of my hospital. These bums take staff and resources away from the people who are really sick."

There had obviously not been time between phone calls for Dr. Bismo to receive a full report on the patient's condition. I decided his Neanderthal view on alcoholism was unchangeable and decided to concentrate on the other medical issues involved. I read him the previous shift's report.

"Now you're a doctor and we're just EMTs," I said. "I admit he was drunk and we may have made a mistake, but even if you were there with us and saw him bleeding, could you have guaranteed us he didn't have any emergency medical problems?"

I was being so nice my stomach was turning. At least the butterflies were gone. I smelled victory.

His tone softened considerably. "Alright, I see your point. Maybe you were right to take him to a hospital; but he's stable now and you can transfer him out."

"I'm sorry, we can't do that," I replied.

"Why not?" he demanded, his voice starting to rise again.

I explained my reasoning to him.

"I don't give a damn about your problems," he stormed. "I want that drunk out of my ER now. I'm the city police surgeon and as such I order you to transfer him out."

Police surgeon? Our city has a police surgeon? I had never seen Dr. Bismo or anyone else for that matter function in that capacity. I'm not calling the man a liar. I'm thoroughly convinced he was paid as our city's police surgeon. I'm simply stating I had never seen Dr. Bismo function as a police surgeon. I wasn't even sure exactly what it was a police surgeon was supposed to do.

Regardless, it was time to play my ace in the hole. I had worked like a dog for this ambulance service for several years. Often I put in 30-35 hours a week, all without pay on top of my full-time job. You see, I was a volunteer. Not only was I a volunteer, but I was also the shift captain and pay day had arrived. A volunteer's only superiors are his line officers. Politicians and hot-headed doctors don't count. My ace in the hole was simply to hold my ground. What could they do, fire me? All the ranting and raving in the world weren't going to help Dr. Bismo.

"I'm sorry doctor," I replied. "I still can't transfer that patient right now."

I could see his bright red face in the telephone and the steam was pouring forth again.

"Let me talk to your superior," he stormed.

Hee hee. "I am the superior."

He was on the run now. There was some stuttering and stammering followed by, "I am also the city coroner and as coroner I'm ordering you to transfer that patient right now."

Coroner? We have a coroner? Why were we transporting all the DOA's first to the hospital for the pronouncement of death by the emergency room physician and then to the funeral home if we have a coroner? I couldn't help wondering how many more unsolicited confessions might be forthcoming.

Anyway, I pleasantly and politely refused his request once again.

The face in the phone turned deep purple and the phone started to melt.

"I'm calling the mayor right now," raged Dr. Bismo.

"Okay," I replied.

He slammed down the phone and mine gradually started to cool as his face faded from the receiver.

I never heard about it again. The mayor knew from experience how fruitless it was to argue with us on such issues. He had learned years ago to just quietly accept the political advantages of supporting a very popular ambulance service - for which he often took credit.

Medical victories in this field are common. Political victories are few and far between. I can count mine on the tip of one finger.

Score one for the good guys.

15. Winter Fun

"What time is it?" Benny called from outside the tent in a trembling voice. "Walt, what time is it?" he repeated.

My eyes reluctantly opened to narrow slits. The pale dim light of early dawn was just beginning to illuminate the tent. I sleepily groped for my watch and held it two inches in front of my still half-closed eyes.

"Six o'clock," I yelled out to Benny.

I closed my eyes again and stuffed myself deeper into my warm sleeping bag. I was almost asleep when the warning bell went off inside my head.

Who cares what time it is? We were out in the middle of nowhere. There was nothing in particular that needed to be done.

Benny didn't need to know what time it was. He wanted to get me up. I didn't know why he wanted me up, but there must be a good reason. I figured I better go find out.

Sometimes things build up and start to get out of hand. You get a streak of bad calls lasting several weeks and you begin to wonder if you're cursed. My favorite way to deal with this is to get away and go camping.

When I say camping, I mean camping. Most of the people I know don't go camping; they go partying out in the woods. They get a large group of people, find a campground with more conveniences than they have in their homes, and have a party.

This is fine with me. I've been to several of these parties and have always had a great time. I simply refuse to call it camping.

First you get a road map. Look for a spot with no large towns nearby and hardly any roads. Then get some topographical maps of this area. These maps will show you the contour of the land and every creek and building in the area. Pick a desolate road, miles from any building. This will be the spot where you're going to leave the car. Then look for a source of running water (stream, river, etc.) at least a few miles from the road. This will be your campsite.

Finally, pack your backpack. Be careful in choosing the items to bring. Remember everything you're going to need for the entire trip will be carried for miles on your back.

This is camping.

When I first asked Benny if he wanted to go along he thought I was kidding. I assured him I was serious. Then he thought I was crazy.

"It's the middle of winter," he protested.

"No problem," I assured him. "I've been winter camping before. We'll build an igloo to sleep in."

I was losing credibility rapidly.

Poor Benny had never been camping before – even in fair weather. I was determined to show him the joys of "real" camping in upper New York State. Every bit of common sense he had told him this idea was ludicrous but in the end my persistence paid off. He looked at me with a look of impending doom in his eyes and nodded approval.

I arranged for him to borrow or buy the best equipment available. I also made sure he had plenty of the right kind of clothes. We studied the menu as I explained the rationale for each of the foods I had selected.

I brought the topographical maps into the station and we picked out our campsite.

Conrad was on station that day and watched intently as I explained the contour lines and symbols on the maps. He decided these maps were the ideal tool for staging war games and he proceeded to do just that with a few of the other guys.

All medics are a bit crazy, but some of us are crazier than others.

Anyway, Benny was starting to get into the swing of things. It looked like he was beginning to lose his initial doubts. At least it looked like that until Conrad slapped him on the back on his way out and proclaimed for the millionth time, "Remember, sometimes you eat the bear and sometimes the bear eats you."

I really wished he hadn't said that.

As the time grew closer it became obvious our trip would encounter a worse climate than I had ever experienced camping. The area of upper New York State we were going to was having temperatures ranging about -15 to -20 F with winds of 30-40 mph.

Benny was desperately trying to worm his way out of the trip but to no avail. I finally pointed out to him that our agreement was in effect a verbal contract and I would sue him for all past, current, and future earnings if he didn't honor it.

He thought about it for quite a while and I was afraid he was going to decide it was worth it.

He did insist on bringing some charcoal lighter to make sure we could start a fire. I assured him it wasn't necessary, but conceded on this point just to prove what a reasonable guy I was.

The big day finally arrived and we left bright and early. When we got there we found a foot of snow waiting for us.

After a two mile hike through a foot of snow with full backpacks I kiddingly asked Benny if he was warmer yet. He didn't even crack a smile. Some people have no sense of humor.

I started a fire and we heated up a quick lunch. Now it was time to build the igloo. People from warmer southern climates probably don't realize there are different kinds of snow. Wet snow packs so well it sometimes packs itself into snowballs as it falls. Dry snow doesn't pack. Bitter cold is usually accompanied by dry snow. We had dry snow.

About the best we could manage was to build the igloo one snowball at a time; and even those little snowballs weren't easy to pack.

After several hours Benny was looking pretty ragged. I re-started the fire and gave him the job of tending it.

As darkness approached it became obvious the igloo would not be completed that night. Therefore, I hurriedly set up the two man nylon mountain tent I had brought along.

I had previously side-stepped Benny's queries when he wanted to know why we needed a tent along. Now he had his answer.

We were both pretty tired so I fixed supper and decided to turn in. Benny said he wanted to play some cards so we played two games of gin rummy. I skunked him both games. It just wasn't his day.

He wanted to continue but I was tired and went to sleep. Actually, I think he was just afraid to go to sleep.

Now he was waking me in the early morning hours to ask what time it was. I quickly dressed and scrambled outside to survey the situation.

Every time I think of that scene now I can't help laughing, but at the time it was too serious and needed prompt action.

Benny was about as blue as I've even seen a live person and shivering like crazy. He must have been trying to start a fire because the fireplace was full of large, only slightly scorched logs. (No kindling in sight.) The precious can of charcoal lighter lay empty on the ground.

You would think he would be appreciative when I rebuilt the fire and started it with only two matches, but his mood seemed to darken still further.

His outlook grew even worse when he realized our eggs were frozen.

I warned him the water wasn't hot enough for hot cocoa yet but he was too impatient. He ended up drinking cold, lumpy, semi-dissolved chocolate water instead of good hot cocoa like mine.

Finally, he informed me he was going home. He gave me three options. The first option was to go with him. The second was to give him the car keys and be left behind. The third option I don't want to talk about.

Since I am such a reasonable person, I decided to elect the first option. After several hours in the car with the heater going full blast, Benny started showing signs of life again.

It is a credit to our friendship that our friendship survived.

However, I don't think Benny has even gone camping again. I guess it was a mistake to make Benny's first camping trip a winter one.

16. Fire

We greeted Nina and Jack as we entered the hospital with our patient. They volunteered for a neighboring town. They were replacing their equipment and were just about ready to leave.

It had been a typically quiet Sunday morning with only a few minor calls. The cold winter air was crisp and clean.

As we left the hospital we heard the fire alarm. We knew it was in Nina and Jack's town and that they were available, so we weren't surprised to hear them acknowledge the call and respond to the initial alarm.

In another minute Jack's voice was on the radio again, requesting more fire department units and a backup ambulance. It sounded serious.

We were nearby and responded immediately.

I still don't know exactly what happened at that taxi garage. A gasoline truck was filling their underground tank. Apparently gasoline was somehow sprayed all over the garage. Something ignited it and the two drivers who were inside became part of the fireball.

A policeman saw them run outside in flames. He knocked them down and threw his coat over them, but didn't roll them or pat it down. When Nina and Jack arrived and took off the coat, they were still on fire.

When Mark and I got there, Nina and Jack already had things pretty well in hand. Both victims were already in the their ambulance and we helped finish applying the burn dressings.

The terrible smell of burnt flesh permeated the air. Our patients had 80-90% third degree burns and one of them was unfortunate enough to still be conscious.

They tell you in class that third degree burns destroy the nerve endings and are therefore painless. This is one of those meaningless facts that has no practical application but that instructors find fascinating. What they usually fail to mention is that third degree burns are surrounded by second degree burns which are extremely painful.

Jack and Nina rushed the patients to the hospital while Mike and I stood by at the fire scene in case of further injuries. The garage burned to the ground.

A little later on we assisted in transporting the patients to the football field for helicopter transport to a burn center.

One of them died that day. The other died several days later.

It was the type of call that continues to haunt us long after it's over; but this one had an ironic twist.

A few months later I responded to a call by the police department for an emotionally disturbed patient. When I got there I found a large man in his early forties throwing cops all over the place. He was wild and totally out of control. Six of us finally managed to bring him to the floor and restrain him.

He passed out for a few minutes and when he came around again he was a completely different person. This had happened to him before so he had a general idea of the commotion he had caused. He apologized profusely and quietly agreed to a hospital evaluation of his emotional state. At that point we couldn't have asked for a nicer or more cooperative patient.

He was the owner of the taxi company.

Over the next couple years we picked him up on several occasions, each one the same. These scenes gave a harsh reality to our own nightmares of screams of pain and burning flesh. They reminded us that we are not the only ones affected by these calls. Most often others are affected even more deeply than we are.

17. DOA

Our patient looked like something you would see in a training film. He was showing every sign and symptom in the book.

His skin was cool, pale and clammy. He was nauseated and had vomited prior to our arrival. His eyes were wide with fear which matched his restless anxiety. The classic crushing chest pain radiating to the left arm was also present.

Our patient was having his first heart attack. Wayne was only 51 years old but there was no doubt about the diagnosis. There was no need for EKG's, blood work or x-rays. The answer was staring us right in the face.

I have witnessed many heart attacks and have noted all possible combinations of the above signs and symptoms. Sometimes a heart attack patient doesn't even have chest pain. They can be very tricky at times and present a true diagnostic challenge.

But when all the signs and symptoms come together like they were now, even a child could make the diagnosis.

We put Wayne on oxygen, recorded his vital signs, carried him downstairs to the ambulance, and raced to the hospital. It was all we could do as a basic life support service.

I tried to contact the hospital on the radio but as usual I was unsuccessful. They kept their radio turned off because they didn't like being interrupted by the "noise".

8:15 Sunday morning saw us wheeling Wayne into a nearly empty emergency room. The staff present consisted of one doctor and one nurse. There were no other patients.

Our patient was still conscious and talking to us as we transferred him to the emergency room cot. As we did so I was giving my report, but it was falling on deaf ears.

The nurse returned to her daily duty of checking out the medicine cabinet while the doctor retreated to his corner to finish the Sunday paper. I guess we had disturbed them.

I was having trouble accepting the way these people were dealing with this obviously acute emergency. I went over to the nurse and mentioned to her quietly that I thought our patient was having a heart attack.

"You're not a doctor," she informed me. "You're not allowed to make a diagnosis."

A glance at the patient from across the room told me he was unconscious now.

"Doctor, I think he stopped breathing," I yelled. "Is he in arrest?"

There was no EKG and no IV in the patient yet. The only treatment he had been given was the oxygen flowing through the mask we had put on him. It was the type of mask with a small plastic oxygen reservoir bag on the bottom.

The doctor went to the head of the cot and looked at Wayne for a few minutes. "I think so," he replied. Then he reached over with his fist from the top of the stretcher and did a kind of drum roll all over Wayne's chest.

Suddenly Nurse Cool had been transformed into Nurse Panic-Stricken. "I'll call the code team!" she yelled at the top of her lungs, running and stumbling toward the call button.

"Relax," barked the doctor. "Take it easy."

"Oh, okay," she replied turning away from the call button to return to her precious medicine cabinet.

On seeing his instructions misinterpreted, the doctor decided to panic now.

"Call the code, call the code," he yelled angrily. "Get over here and do CPR."

Nurse Panic returned to the call button and I immediately heard the speakers announce: "Code Blue – ER, Code Blue – ER, Code Blue – ER."

The official notification of the Code was documented at 8:28 A.M. The termination of the code was ordered by the ER doctor and documented at 8:39 A.M. This was the same time listed on the death certificate. It was documented on the line right under the letters D.O.A. (dead on arrival).

In those eleven minutes the doctor first attempted to ventilate the patient by squeezing the little plastic reservoir bag on the bottom of the face mask.

"You're not doing any good," I yelled at the doctor.

"Yes, I'm squeezing the bag, see?" he answered.

"Where's the bag-mask resuscitator?" I demanded.

Neither one of them knew where it was. I ran out to the ambulance to get ours but by then the code team had arrived with their own (I guess they didn't know where the ER kept it either).

They started the IV and got the EKG hooked up. The doctor ordered sodium bicarbonate to treat the developing acidosis.

That was it.

No cardiac medications were given. No electric shock was administered.

The doctor walked across the hallway to the relatives who had arrived in the interim. He told the relatives who had seen us carry their loved one out of the house conscious and talking, that he was dead on arrival.

In all fairness to the doctor, this was official hospital policy. You see, Wayne hadn't been admitted to the hospital yet. If he wasn't admitted, he couldn't have died there so he must have been D.O.A.

D.O.A. Those three letters did more to keep that hospital's mortality rate low than any medical treatment they ever gave.

18. Teddy Bear

It was a hot summer day and my sweat was dripping all over our patient as I strained to lift her wheelchair up through the side door of our ambulance.

"Why the hell doesn't Larry put a hydraulic life on one of these things?" I wondered to myself for the thousandth time.

"Look at the way you're sweating," our patient said. "It's too hot to be working like this today."

This was Jennie, one of our very special patients – one of many.

Jennie was a kidney dialysis patient. Three times a week we took her to the regional dialysis center where she spent the day hooked up to tubes and needles. Without maintaining this strict regimen, she would die.

The rest of her life was spent maintaining a very strict diet of pills and unappetizing food. Like many dialysis patients, Jennie also suffered from numerous other maladies related to her kidney problems.

The future for a dialysis patient, who is not a candidate for transplant, holds the promise of increased problems and suffering followed by death.

I don't know how these people manage to survive, but many of them maintain a better outlook than a lot of healthy people I know. I guess that's the only thing that really matters.

I secured Jennie's wheelchair and hopped into my seat. Jim reached for the ignition to start the ambulance, but Jennie stopped him.

"Wait a minute, Jim," she said, reaching into her bag. "I've got something for you."

She pulled out a little teddy bear she had crocheted and handed it to Jim with a smile.

I watched Jim's face intently to see what his reaction would be.

All of us at Central Ambulance Service had received a teddy bear from Jennie except Joe. He was our newest medic. We had them sitting all over our office in Bergenfield, New Jersey. We also kept one in every ambulance where they came in very handy.

On more than one occasion these bears had helped to calm a nervous pediatric patient.

Even more importantly, though, we had discovered that by playing with these bears very conspicuously as we drove through some of the rougher neighborhoods of New York City, we could avoid being harassed as we had been on many previous trips. No one wants to mess with a crazy man - and if you're a grown man conspicuously playing with teddy bears in a rough neighborhood - well, you had to be crazy.

Jim just stared at Jennie blankly for a second or two. Then, slowly, a smile came to his face.

"Aw gee, thanks Jennie," he said. "He's adorable."

I breathed a sigh of relief. It was over at last. Jim was no longer a rookie.

This may seem like a strange way to judge rookie status, but Jim was a kind of strange guy.

I've never found a time limit or a level of achievement to be useful for judging rookie status. In my book, you're a rookie until you stop acting like one. This may be a rather subjective definition, but it's always worked for me.

Actually, Jim was already an experienced medic when Lou hired him. It really didn't matter though; he was still a rookie with us. He probably could have shed his rookie status pretty quickly. He was a big, strong, hardworking man and he was a good medic. He only had one problem. He didn't like being considered a rookie. The more he didn't like it, the more we considered him one.

Things had gotten pretty bad. Jim felt he had to prove how tough he was so we wouldn't walk all over him.

During one of our typical arguments a few days ago he had fixed me with a cold hard stare and blurted out, "I'm going to rip your heart out and hand it to you before you die."

I laughed so hard tears were rolling down my cheeks, "That's a great line," I told him. "Do you mind if I borrow it sometime?"

Jim just hung his head and walked away, beaten.

Hollywood must have thought it was a great line, too, because years later they borrowed the concept in the filming of *Indiana Jones and the Temple of Doom*. I don't think Jim ever got any royalties.

Now, as I watched the smile on his face, I knew the struggle was over. Jim's tough guy image would never have allowed him to accept the teddy bear so graciously.

Jim went on to become one of the principal employees of Central Ambulance Service, but I've always wondered what would have happened if Jennie hadn't made that teddy bear for him.

We'll always remember you, Jennie.

19. The Little Room

My palms weren't just sweaty, they were dripping. My whole body was a bundle of nerves. I went to the bathroom. Ten minutes later I had to go again.

The bathroom was getting quite a workout that day. I was not alone. There were fifteen other paramedic students waiting to be tested for our final practical exam.

With six years of ambulance experience it shouldn't have been this hard. I had started as a mere first-aider. From there I had earned my EMT certification. I went on to become an EMT instructor. Now I was working in Indiana and at the end of my paramedic course; the highest level of training available for pre-hospital care. Ten long months of intensive study and clinical rotation were behind me.

The setup was simple. There were four stations located in four different rooms. In each one a different individual skill or combination of skills would be tested.

Jack, our instructor, was a nice guy. He was a big man who for some reason always reminded me of a walrus. Jack was a paramedic himself, one of the best. His classes had taught us not only the book knowledge, but as much as possible, the field applications as well.

The ever present smile on his face went along with his willingness to go out of his way to help anyone he could in any way he could.

There's only one other thing you need to know about Jack. He would kick anyone out of the course at any time without hesitation if that person failed to maintain the high standards prescribed at the beginning of the course.

We all knew medics who had survived ten long months of arduous study only to flunk out on the final written or practical test. The word was if you passed Joe's course, the state licensure test was a breeze.

As a matter of fact, no one who graduated from Jack's course had ever flunked the state exam.

Now it was my turn. The stations were all graded on a pass/fail system. I had to pass them all. There would be no second chance. A failure would require repeating the expense and the work of the entire course – or giving up my dream. I wasn't sure which option I would pick.

I was third in line waiting to get into The Little Room. The Little Room was the worst station of all. It had been the downfall of more medics than any other part of the course.

I knew what to expect inside. Jack would be inside The Little Room with a slide projector and a screen. He would flash fifteen slides of EKG's – one at a time. Each one would be shown for only fifteen seconds. After fifteen seconds I would be required to give the heart rate and rhythm interpretation, state whether or not treatment would be required, and if so what the treatment would be.

The passing criteria was simple. It required no mathematics to figure out your score. If you missed one it was over.

It seemed like the guys in front of me were taking hours. I tried to review EKG's in my mind, but I was too nervous and gave up. If I didn't know them by now, it was too late to learn.

My classmates looked very pale and uncertain of themselves as one by one they exited The Little Room. We wouldn't be told the results until the next day.

I started considering what other career I might be good at. I couldn't think of any.

The guy in front of me disappeared into The Little Room. The room seemed to gobble him up as the door closed. I was next.

The pressure was unbearable. Now I knew why they required a physical exam before starting the course. Anyone with a heart condition could die of a heart attack here.

This guy was taking forever in there. What was Jack doing to him?

Finally the door opened and he stumbled out on rubbery legs.

"Next," Jack called from inside. I considered running away.

I stepped in and shut the door behind me. The walls immediately started to close in around me. This really was a little room. I was certain there was a puddle of sweat at my feet.

Jack made some small talk in an attempt to relax me, but the glazed look in my eyes told him it was as useless as it had been with the rest.

"Alright, let's get on with it," he said flashing the first slide.

I looked at it and thought, "ventricular tachycardia".

It can't be that simple, there must be a trick. I had only about ten seconds left to find out what the trick was. I stared at it like I had never seen an EKG before. I couldn't find anything else.

Darkness enveloped the room as the slide disappeared in front of my eyes. "Ventricular tachycardia at a rate of 180/minute," I said, my voice cracking. "Check for a pulse. If no pulse, start CPR and cardiovert at 200 joules. If a pulse is present but the patient is unresponsive, cardiovert at 200 joules. If the patient is conscious give lidocaine IV push 1 milligram/kilogram and repeat at 0.5 milligram/kilogram if necessary up to a maximum of 200 milligrams. Then start a lidocaine drip with a 4:1 concentration at 2-4 milligrams/minute."

"Okay, next," Joe said. I knew he wouldn't tell me if I was right but he seemed satisfied.

The next strip also looked easy. I wondered what I was missing as I blurted out the interpretation and treatment.

"Okay, next," Joe said and flashed another slide.

We went through thirteen more of those slides in similar fashion. When it was over Jack turned on the lights and asked me to send the next student in.

I couldn't resist the urge to ask him how I had done.

Jack looked at me and grinned. "How do you think you did?" was all he would say.

The EKG's really hadn't been all that difficult. The pressure was obviously manufactured just for us.

I left The Little Room cursing Jack's previously unrecognized sadistic nature.

Five months later I was kneeling on the floor next to my patient with a crisp new paramedic patch on the right sleeve of my uniform shirt.

I had passed all the stations of the practical test – even The Little Room. My final grade average was 95%, comfortably above the 80% needed to pass and the second best in my class. The hospital and field preceptors had submitted good reports on my performance.

After all that, the state's written and practical exam did almost seem easy - I passed with the highest score in my class.

One final physical exam required by the state proved I had survived my training with sufficient health to perform the duties of a paramedic.

Now I was busy trying to estimate the amount of blood on the floor between my patient's legs.

My 25-year-old patient had delivered a baby one week ago. When she started hemorrhaging vaginally her neighbor, who was visiting, called us right away.

She was white as a sheet and was very lethargic. Her blood pressure was 60/0 and her radial pulse was imperceptible. I put the MAST (Medical Anti-Shock Trousers) on and inflated them while my partner was setting up an IV for me. I had learned in class that MAST works by shunting the blood away from the lower extremities and up to the head and chest where it is needed most.

Now I had to start the IV. The ironic thing about IV's is that they're the most difficult to start when you need them the most. I wanted to put two large bore IV's in my patient to run in lots of fluid, but the veins were flat because of the blood loss and it wouldn't be easy.

Suddenly, as I knelt on the floor bent over my patient, I became aware of two small legs standing next to me. I looked up into the tearful face of a sobbing six-year-old girl.

"Please save my mommy," she begged. In the next room I could hear the week old infant wailing as if he knew what was happening too.

"I'll do my best," I assured her.

Then I shut her out of my mind. I couldn't afford to see or hear her anymore.

Some of you may think having your boss look over your shoulder while you're working is pressure. I don't care if your boss is eight feet tall, weighs 400 pounds, has claws a foot long, and a single eye in the middle of his forehead. He can't come close to putting the type of pressure on you that this little six-year-old was putting on me.

I got two IV's going and ran in the Ringer's Lactate IV Solution as fast as I could. They were 16 gauge IV needles – the ones so big they could sometimes leave small scars.

My patient started to improve as I transported her. I was relieved when the doctor told me she would be okay.

Several months later I bumped into her as I was leaving the emergency room. She was at the hospital visiting a friend. She made a point of showing me the scars the IV's had left in her arms. I thought she was mad but then she smiled and thanked me. She told me her doctor had informed her that I had saved her life.

I walked away glowing with pride and reflecting on the call. While I was reflecting on it, I recalled the intense pressure the little girl had inadvertently subjected me to.

Out of the blue, memories of The Little Room popped into my head.

Suddenly, I understood the purpose of The Little Room. The Little Room wasn't a test of EKG knowledge. All the knowledge in the world wouldn't help if we couldn't function under pressure.

If we were going to crack under pressure, Jack wanted it to happen right there in The Little Room; not out in the field when someone's life would be hanging in the balance.

As always Jack was doing his best to assure our welfare and the welfare of our future patients.

20. Jet Ski

The teenager lying before me on the lounge chair didn't look so bad. Not while he was lying on his back, anyway.

He was playing around on a jet ski in the lake of this exclusive neighborhood. Some horsing around had caused a fall and when he surfaced again he was struggling.

Fortunately there were some quick thinking Good Samaritans around. They took a lounge chair out into the lake, submerged it under him, and lifted him out with it.

The reason they all looked kind of green and sickly now was the sight they were greeted with when they went out to rescue the kid.

Sometime during the fall the kid had lacerated his back and when he did, his intestines popped out, protruding from the wound.

Now, as he lay unconscious in front of me, I planned my course of action. Sylvia and I had to assume he had spinal injuries until x-rays at the hospital proved otherwise.

His blood pressure and pulse were high. I knew in a teenager this meant they were compensating for significant blood loss. If left untreated, his body would no longer be able to compensate and he would develop a possibly irreversible and lethal state of shock.

103

His respiratory status was adequate and according to his rescuers he had never stopped breathing.

One of the bystanders stepped forward and identified himself as a doctor. Upon questioning him I found out he was an eye doctor. Regardless, I had him start an IV in one arm while I started one in the other. I was glad he did because his was running in faster than mine. The lost blood had to be replaced with an increased circulating volume.

When the dressing, bandage, sterile saline, and spineboard were ready, we log-rolled the kid onto his side carefully keeping his head, neck, and spine aligned.

That's when I saw his evisceration for the first time. His intestines had bulged out and covered the laceration hiding it from sight.

I covered them with a large trauma dressing soaked with normal saline. This would keep them from drying out and help prevent further contamination. Then we rolled him onto his back again onto the spineboard with MAST in place.

The intestines were at the small of his back so lying supine did not put excessive pressure on them. We zipped up the inflatable trousers but did not inflate them yet. With his blood pressure still elevated, he didn't need them yet, but I wanted them ready at a moment's notice if he should take a sudden turn for the worse.

We took our patient to the rig, switched from the portable oxygen tank to the main line, and hooked up the EKG so we could monitor his heart rate easier.

His heart rate and blood pressure were dropping slowly. A sudden precipitous drop in blood pressure with a rising pulse would have signaled a life – threatening worsening in his condition. This slow drop in both blood pressure and pulse, however, was an improvement showing a return to normal.

He was also starting to show signs of regaining consciousness. This helped ease my worries about a possible head injury and Sylvia and I started to breathe easier.

From the ER he was rushed to surgery. Following that was some intensive IV antibiotic therapy. In a few weeks he was home with only a scar to show for his traumatic adventure.

I'm not sure if he ever went jet skiing again, but at least I never had to treat him again.

21. Scarred

"You're vile and disgusting!" Tina shouted as she ran from the room. Sammy and I just looked at each other.

"What got into her?" he asked.

We were discussing the similarities between the topping on the pizza in front of us and the brains we had just seen splattered across the front end of a car.

"I don't know," I replied.

We both did know, of course. It was time to have a talk with our new rookie.

When I was a rookie, someone told me that you get as cold as steel in this business. He said you reach a point where nothing bothers you.

Bullshit.

That never happened to me and I never wanted it to. I've only seen it happen to a couple guys and when it did they became useless and had to leave. There's no room for that type of attitude in this field. We do need to learn how to turn it off at the scene. There's no time for that and we can't afford an emotional response at that time. After the call is over, it's a different story.

106

Actually, you end up tiptoeing along a very fine line. Without the caring, compassion, and a little self-doubt, you lose your desire to improve or even to be in this field at all.

But if you step over the line you can destroy yourself. Your doubts and worries and stress build to a point where they incapacitate you.

It's quite a balancing act. Sometimes we maintain balance with quiet introspection. Sometimes we need to talk. Other times we make jokes (i.e. pizza). We may escape with physical or mental activity. Shouting and crying are certainly not unheard of.

Different methods work for different people at different times. Overall we get pretty good at our balancing act on most calls.

Not all calls.

Every seasoned EMT and paramedic has had those kind of calls. You hate them. You never want another one. You spend days on end trying to forget the call, but the harder you try, the more vividly the details become etched in your memory.

Finally you realize it's happened again and give up trying to forget. You've been scarred again – deeper and more horribly than any switchblade could ever do. Scarred for life by a memory that will never go away and that will bring tears to your eyes and a lump to your throat every time you think about it.

You hate it – but in a strange and unexplainable way you need it, too. It becomes part of who you are.

No single mistake could have resulted in such tragedy. The series of misfortunes started a couple a weeks before we got the call.

Joan had a cold. There's nothing unusual about this in a nine-year-old girl. However, when her condition worsened and she progressed to pneumonia, her parents failed to recognize it as a problem. They were very ignorant of medical care so they weren't concerned that she had vomiting and diarrhea for days while being unable to eat or drink. They weren't aware of the dangers of dehydration, electrolyte imbalance, and malnutrition.

The first time they realized something was wrong was when they couldn't awaken Joan after she "fell asleep" on the floor. Their reaction was not to call us, but to call their volunteer fire department.

Any fire department in the world would have called us immediately except this one. They were going to prove they could handle a sick child as well as those hotshot paramedics with all their fancy equipment.

They found Joan in cardiac arrest when they got there. They decided they better call us.

When Bill and I got there we found the fire department doing chest compressions. Not CPR – chest compressions. CPR includes mouth-to-mouth ventilations. They were not ventilating her. Joan had vomited.

It is not easy to do mouth-to-mouth ventilation on someone who has vomited. Believe me, I am an expert on this subject and I know. I also know that compressions by themselves are useless and that your patient will die if you don't do mouth-to-mouth.

We started mouth-to-mouth ventilations while getting our fancy equipment ready.

Her pupils were fixed and dilated; usually a sign of brain death. Her heart showed no electrical activity at all on our monitor – another very poor prognostic sign.

I cleared her airway and passed an endotracheal tube down her windpipe to protect her airway and to ventilate her better. I started an IV and pushed all of the drugs allowed under these circumstances by my standing protocol orders. Sodium bicarbonate, epinephrine, atropine.

Nothing.

I administered an electric shock to the heart in case the monitor was misleading me and there was slight electrical activity I couldn't see.

Nothing.

Radio contact was made with the hospital. I wanted further orders.

Once you've used up protocol orders and need more, the doctor on the other end of the radio can make the difference between life and death. I've seen it work both ways.

When he heard the nature of the call, the doctor got on the radio himself. This is unusual. Normally they communicate through a nurse.

His voice was also unusual. I had never heard it before. He was new to our hospital's staff and I didn't even know who he was.

It didn't matter. I liked him. The orders came snapping over the radio – clear, precise, logical.

I followed them. Calcium chloride, an isuprel drip.

Nothing.

We had a 40 minute transport time to the hospital. For all practical purposes, Joan was going to live or die right here. I wanted to do more.

"Rescue 9 requesting orders for 50% dextrose," I radioed in.

"Does your patient have any history of diabetes?" asked the doctor.

"Negative – no known history. But maybe it wasn't diagnosed – and she could probably use the sugar anyway," I replied.

I was reaching for straws now.

"Go ahead with the dextrose and also push an amp of narcan."

Narcan? In case of narcotic overdose? Well, it wouldn't hurt and one straw is as good as another. I followed the orders.

Nothing.

My bag of tricks was empty. We got the order to transport.

While enroute to the hospital, my monitor started beeping. A cardiac rhythm had appeared. The isuprel drip must have kicked in. I checked for a pulse. Joan had strong pulses!

I checked for spontaneous respirations.

Nothing.

I checked the pupils.

Still fixed and dilated.

We had successfully resuscitated the heart, even after all the abuse it had received. But the brain had been without oxygen for too long.

Seven years of experience couldn't help me now. Her brain was dead – and so was Joan.

22. Dr. Anderson

"Dr. Muckson has confirmed the order," the ER nurse informed us over the radio. "Give 100 milligrams of lidocaine IV push NOW." The emphasis was on the last word.

This was one of those notorious EMS career killers – also known as being caught between a rock and a hard place.

I checked my patient again. She still had a very slow pulse and the EKG monitor was still showing an idioventricular rhythm; a slow abnormal heart beat that just barely keeps the heart going when everything else has failed.

Lidocaine is supposed to knock out ventricular rhythms; specifically extra beats or fast ventricular rhythms. Then the normal rhythm of the heart can resume. In this case, there was no normal rhythm to take over. If I knocked out the idioventricular rhythm the patient would die.

At least, that's what I had been taught. That's also what I had read in every related medical book and article I had seen. My understanding of the mechanism of lidocaine and the electrophysiology of the heart also led me to the same conclusion.

But what if I'm wrong? Dr. Muckson is, after all, a doctor with a great deal more training and experience than I have.

Just a few short minutes ago this had been a very serious but rather routine ambulance call. Now I was faced with a plethora of medical, legal, and moral complexities.

The law has never been clear to me on any matter. My best guess based on hypothetical arguments with instructors and lawyers is that I have to do what is right for the patient. If the doctor gives me an inappropriate order, he can get into trouble. If I follow that order and I should have known better, I also get into trouble. If I refuse to follow an order because I believe it is inappropriate and it turns out it was correct, I get into trouble again.

In other words, there is no room for error. Regardless of who gave the order my decision has to be correct or I am legally responsible for the consequences.

Medically and morally the picture is even worse. If any decision is correct, the patient might live. The wrong decision will kill the patient.

Whether I am right or wrong, refusing a doctor's orders is not the ideal way to maintain a good working relationship.

Did I have enough faith in Dr. Muckson to follow his order blindly and contradict everything I had learned, read and could understand?

No. This patient was not going to get lidocaine. Not from me, anyway.

While my partner prepared her for transport, I got on the radio and repeated my objections to the order. The argument continued enroute to the hospital. Dr. Muckson was adamant, but my stubbornness was too much for him and he finally gave up.

The atmosphere when we got to the ER wasn't exactly friendly, but frankly I had expected worse.

The patient survived and Dr. Muckson never did file charges against me. I filed an incident report to determine the right answer conclusively. I was assured that my decision was correct and my reasoning was sound.

To my knowledge Dr. Muckson was never informed of this. The exact same problem was repeated at least twice with other medics.

Actually, things have improved dramatically in the last 14 years. The advent of the American College of Emergency Physicians has gone a long way toward improving the emergency care of patients.

Prior to this many emergency rooms were staffed with any doctor the administration could find. This often included obstetricians, radiologists, anesthesiologists, family practice physicians wanting to build up their own practice, and semi-retired doctors who wanted to keep their hand in medicine to a limited extent. Sometimes it even included physicians being reprimanded by the hospital's administrator.

Some of these made good emergency physicians, but overall they left much to be desired. You don't want a cardiologist treating your broken bones, a surgeon treating your diabetes, or a general practitioner treating your heart attack. You want an emergency medicine specialist treating your medical emergency.

The transition to emergency medicine specialists is still in the infant stage, but the trend is in the right direction.

The trend was started by doctors like Dr. Anderson.

Ten years ago when our nearest hospital closed, we started bringing some of our patients to Savior Hospital. After several years of battling with apathetic ER physicians, I had strayed from what I knew was the proper treatment for my patients.

The treatment we could give in the field was very limited at that time. We were supposed to record the vitals of every patient, but this would only be helpful if the ER staff used the vitals we took to compare with their own. In this way they could determine the stability of the patient.

The ER staffs we dealt with barely managed to take their own vitals and couldn't care less about our assessment. Therefore, I reasoned, it was a waste of time to take vitals in the field. The patient would be better served by using the time to transport instead.

At least, that's what I believed until I ran into a buzz saw by the name of Dr. Anderson.

The first time I met him I was bringing a patient with only minor injuries into his ER.

"Why didn't you call in a report on the radio?" he demanded gruffly.

"The hospitals always leave their radios turned off so the noise won't bother them," I replied.

"In my hospital when I'm on duty the radio is <u>never</u> turned off," he said his voice rising in anger. "What are your patient's vitals?"

My jaw dropped open and I stood there with a dumbfounded look on my face. I didn't know.

I wouldn't have believed this tall thin 65-year-old man topped by a balding white scalp could frighten me but his glasses were steaming up and he looked like he was about to jump down my throat.

He chewed my ass good and ended it with a warning to never bring a patient to his ER again unless I had done my job properly.

A few weeks later I arrived at Dr. Anderson's ER again. I beamed with pride as I gave him a full report following my earlier radio report on my patient. I stood there with a stupid grin on my face waiting for a compliment.

"Well, what are you waiting for?" Dr. Anderson asked. "Do you think you deserve a medal? All you did was to do your job. You should have been doing it all along. No one gives me a medal for doing my job and no one is going to give you one either."

He was right of course. I decided to never allow someone else's incompetence to drag me down again. I would do my best on every call from then on and if other people weren't interested in doing the same that would be their problem. I would not be the weak link in the chain.

23. Seizures

Of all the medical ailments I have treated, seizures present the greatest opportunity for saving a patient in the field.

I'm not talking about saving the patient from the seizure. I'm talking about saving the patient from the well-intentioned bystanders who come to his "aid".

Many seizure patients need no immediate medical treatment. If you are present when someone experiences a seizure you can help the patient to the ground to prevent a head injury from a fall. If they are thrashing about you should remove any nearby objects which could injure them. Call an ambulance just to make sure this is only a simple seizure. When they pass out you can turn them on their side and open the airway as you're taught to do in CPR classes. As they slowly regain consciousness you can quietly and calmly reassure them. This is all that is required for the vast majority or seizure patients.

<u>Do Not Shove Anything In Their Mouth!</u>

I could fill a museum with the assortment of objects I have removed from the mouths of my seizure patients. They include spoons, forks, blocks of wood, dirty socks, and basically anything else within arm's reach that can be jammed into the mouth.

They have resulted in numerous lacerations and broken teeth and could be potentially lethal as sources of hemorrhagic aspiration and airway blockage.

DO NOT SHOVE ANYTHING IN THEIR MOUTH!

The old wives' tale about swallowing the tongue just isn't true. The tongue is attached to the rear of the pallet and cannot be swallowed. It can fall back over the airway, temporarily blocking it. You can relieve this by turning your patient on his side and using the airway maneuvers taught in CPR classes.

Poor Gene was lucky he survived that night.

Gene was a university student living in one of the dorms a few blocks from our station.

We got the first call about 10 PM. Gene's fellow dorm residents had set up a human chain from the sidewalk to his room so we could find it quickly, I was impressed.

They urged us to hurry along the way and warned us that he had turned blue.

This is common in seizure patients. Of course, it was probably worsened by the fact that the 20 people standing around in the small dorm room had used up all the oxygen.

We started throwing people out until we could see our patient. He was unconscious, apparently in what is known as a typical post-ictal state.

Kneeling at his side was his roommate. He was holding a steak knife in Gene's mouth. Fortunately he had the handle end in his mouth.

His roommate explained that he couldn't find a spoon or fork so he had to use a knife. His own hand had been lacerated from holding the blade end of the knife and at this point I wasn't sure which of them needed our attention more.

Carefully I withdrew the knife from Gene's mouth. Then I bandaged his roommate's hand.

During the ride to the hospital I admonished the roommate for his actions and pointed out to him that any hard object placed in a seizing patient's mouth could cause trauma to the mouth.

He seemed to understand.

Gene recovered from the seizure and after some blood tests was discharged from the hospital a few hours later.

The second call came in at 1:30 AM. Gene had seized again.

We found the network to guide us to the room in place again. This time the crowd parted as we entered so we didn't have to fight like Chicago defensive linemen trying to sack a quarterback.

Gene was unconscious again. There was nothing sticking out of his mouth, but his cheeks looked suspiciously bloated. I opened his mouth and withdrew a greenish-yellow scuzzy looking handkerchief. I held it up by one corner and gave his roommate a questioning look.

"I have a cold," he said.

My frustration got the better of me.

"DO NOT SHOVE ANYTHING IN HIS MOUTH!!!" I yelled.

He cowered in the corner with a hurt puppy dog look on his face.

A few hours later Gene was discharged from the hospital again. Apparently they REALLY believed seizures were no big deal.

The third call came in at 5:10 AM. This time the network to show us the way was absent. We knew the way as well as they did by now.

The familiar crowd was out in the hall. Only Gene and his roommate were in the room.

There was nothing sticking out of Gene's mouth and his cheeks weren't bulging. I opened his mouth and searched in it meticulously for about a minute with my penlight.

"Nothing in his mouth?" I inquired of his roommate.

"Nothing in his mouth," he replied nervously.

"Well done," I said smiling reassuringly.

He smiled back beaming with pride.

Just when we finally got it right the hospital finally decided to admit Gene.

DO NOT SHOVE ANYTHING IN THEIR MOUTH!!!

24. More Seizures

Not all seizures patients are as easy to care for as Gene. A small minority of patients can experience prolonged or rapidly repetitive seizures which can be serious and even fatal. Some seizures are caused by other medical problems which can be rapidly lethal if left untreated. That's why an ambulance should be called for every seizure even though it probably won't be necessary for most.

Very rarely a patient is seen who exhibits wild and violent thrashing of his body instead of the relatively innocuous spasms characteristic of most grand mal seizures.

A few patients have taken a swing at me and then tried to get away with it by faking one of these seizures. Unfortunately for them there is a world of difference between a true violent seizure and the somewhat grade F performance they put on. I was neither fooled nor amused.

Felix, however, was for real. From the first time I saw his seizure there was never a doubt in my mind about that.

The first time I saw him he showed all the signs of a true seizure in the postictal state. He was unconscious with snoring respirations and saliva drooling profusely from his mouth. He had soiled his pants and was unresponsive to my prodding and calling him – all signs of a seizure.

What surprised me was his broken arm, numerous bruises and contusions, and the busted furniture all around.

His family warned us that he experienced repetitive seizures which are always very violent. The evidence was there, but I had never seen a seizure that violent and was not yet totally convinced.

By the time we had our stretcher ready, Fernando was starting to come around.

I talked to him softly, answering his repeated questions over and over again until his mind was functioning well enough to begin to comprehend what had happened.

At first he refused transport to the hospital, but as he became more aware of the pain in his broken arm (which we had splinted while he was still unconscious) it became easier to change his mind.

He tried to stand up and when he did all hell broke loose. Felix started the wildest and most violent seizing I have ever seen.

His movements weren't purposeful; he wasn't aiming at anyone or anything, but if you happened to be in the way of his flailing arms, legs, or head it hurt plenty.

Most of the damage Felix was doing, however, was to himself. In the small confined room we were in it was impossible to move things out of his way. Walls don't move easily.

I made a carefully timed lunge for Felix and managed to get in close, past his swinging arms and legs. I threw my arms around him and drew him to me, effectively tying him up. At such close range, the movement of his arms and legs was restricted and not nearly as forceful as they had been.

When he passed out we strapped him to the stretcher and rushed to the hospital.

Felix was still unconscious when we got there. I told the nurse about his seizures and asked if she wanted us to stay around to help.

She smiled at me somewhat amused to find me making such a big deal over a little seizure and assured me that she could handle it.

As we were walking out the door I heard her scream for help.

A smile crossed my lips as I thought it over for a fraction of a second before turning to go back in.

25. CPR

Bruce and I sprinted to the ambulance. The tires screeched as we barely cleared the opening garage door. I knew the odds were heavily against us and from the way Bruce was driving, he knew it too.

The quavering voice in the telephone was still ringing in my ears.

"Hurry, my baby's dying," he had pleaded.

We were hurrying.

I have always firmly believed in doing my best on every call. By always doing your best it becomes routine. Then when you need your best, it comes easily.

Therefore, I believe in driving the same way to every emergency call. Driving faster than this unacceptably increases the risk to us and other drivers.

I firmly believe in this. My mind tells me it is the only rational approach. I want to follow these guidelines – but a baby is dying!

My mind loses it total control and is ruled by a mixture of logic and emotions. It is wrong. It is dangerous to both myself and others. It is a sign of weakness. I know this and I strongly urge others to avoid it. Despite this I have never been able to completely control it. All I can do is keep trying and pray no one gets injured.

Bruce was having the same problem now as we darted through the downtown rush hour traffic.

Our destination was six miles away. The brain dies in four to six minutes without oxygen. It was an impossible task.

Our luck held and we arrived without incident. We flew through the door and found a distraught father administering CPR to his eleven-month-old son.

This is rare. It is so rare we hadn't even considered the possibility.   The odds had just improved considerably.

Little Johnny's color was good and his pupils were still reacting to my penlight. I took over CPR and we raced back to the hospital at a slightly less frenzied pace. At least we now knew Johnny was receiving medical attention.

The doctor was able to resuscitate Johnny in the ER. He was admitted to the hospital to find out what had caused his cardiac arrest. He was transferred to a pediatric hospital and about two months later he was home with his family again. Johnny suffered no lasting effects from his close call with death.

His father's fortuitous choice to take a CPR class several months earlier had been made on a whim. He had no idea at the time that his choice would spell the difference between life and death for his infant son. Johnny's parents thanked us profusely for saving their son's life – but we were the wrong ones to thank. Johnny's dad made the difference on that call.

Joan, Johnny, and a few dozen other adult and pediatric patients just like them led me to the realization a few years later that I hadn't been doing enough.

Of all the patients in cardiac arrest I had treated, only eight had received CPR from the beginning of their cardiac arrest. Four of them went home from the hospital, a percentage equal to any in the nation and an impressive feat when you consider these people were dead to begin with.

The problem was the dozens who were in cardiac arrest before my arrival and were not receiving CPR. Time ran out for them before I could reach them.

I decided just treating patients wasn't enough. It was also my obligation to share my knowledge and skills with the public.

My wife looked at me like I was nuts when I informed her I wanted to register in a CPR instructor course. After nine years of full time ambulance duty, I had switched to another medical career for full time work. I continued to work sixteen hours/week on ambulance, however, which necessitated an additional 60 hours/year of in-service training to keep my paramedic license current. Numerous other obligations further contributed to keeping me away from my wife and baby girl much more than I liked.

Teresa saw the familiar half-crazed look in my eyes and once again nodded her approval for my latest scheme. Her love and understanding are phenomenal.

When I finished my instructor's training I searched for some way to arouse the interest of my audience. A room of half-hearted students who would never use the skills I was trying to teach would not suffice. There had to be a way to motivate them.

There was only one way I could think of to highlight the difference people can make. I decided to tell my classes of my experience with Joan and Johnny. Their reactions surprised me.

These people had never seen Joan or Johnny. Yet the stories brought tears to their eyes. I could see their compassion and their desire to make a difference. This was what had been missing.

I believe the medical profession's most tragic failure has been its inability to motivate and educate the public. All the wondrous machines, miracle drugs, and exhaustive research can't produce a fraction of the results that public education and preventative medicine can.

CPR classes include instruction on prudent heart living –
how to avoid risk factors that can lead to heart disease. We
also teach people how to recognize the warning signs of
impending cardiac arrest and what to do about it. The earlier
you start to deal with a problem, the easier it is to deal with.

There is no one on earth who can't spend one or two
days learning how to save the life of a stranger, a neighbor,
or a loved one. Going to the doctor for a checkup once a
year, just isn't enough.

The big difference will come only when the public
accepts some of the responsibility for their own health and
well-being.

26. Heroes

"South station from central station," the voice on the radio crackled. It had not been preceded by the customary emergency tones. "Could you ask officer 32 to report to central station on his way home?"

I was officer 32. What now? I couldn't think of anything I had done that would get me into trouble. Not in the last 24 hours, anyway.

"Congratulations," George said as we crossed paths at central's front door. "Why didn't you ask? I would have worked for you."

"Congratulations for what?" I replied. "Why did I need someone to work for me?"

"Always a kidder," George responded with a smile as he left.

Denny, the on-coming shift captain greeted me with a handshake. "Here it is. We would have arranged coverage for you if you had asked."

He was pushing a plaque and an envelope in to my hands. The plaque had all the typical words on it like "Paramedic of the Year" and "Outstanding Service". It also had my name on it.

"What's it for?" I asked.

"The citation inside explains everything; but didn't Ted tell you about it?" Denny asked.

Ted was my shift captain. He was supposed to tell me about it so I could be present at the commission meeting to accept it in person.

To this day I don't know if he honestly forgot to tell me or if it was his way of retaliating for the innumerable practical jokes I had subjected him to.

Anyway, I was busy assembling a mental list of my calls from the last year to figure out which one had earned me this honor.

I had received some minor battery acid burns on my face while crawling into a ditch to rescue a patient from an over-turned car, but I didn't think that was it. Crawling under the car was nothing unusual and the burns were very minor. Besides, that patient died a few days later and they generally don't give you awards when your patient dies.

I had delivered a baby on Father's Day that year, but it was the seventh delivery of my career. Delivering babies had never merited an award before.

There were numerous patients I had helped as well as some I had lost. None that I could remember were unusual enough to prompt a citation.

I opened the envelope to satisfy my rapidly increasing curiosity. The citation explained it all.

It said I was on standby at the scene of a house fire when a fireman collapsed on the roof. Despite the presence of the raging fire, I had gone up on the roof without waiting for protective gear and rescued the fireman.

Oh, that call.

Have you ever been told a story that is absolutely true and completely misleading?

The fire was confined to a different part of the house when I made my ascent to the roof. The fireman was suffering only from heat exhaustion and was in pretty good shape when I got to him. He had already regained consciousness and the biggest thing I did for him was to remove his heavy fire coat. He ended up climbing down the ladder himself over my protests – and did it much better than I did. He didn't even go to the hospital.

Still, it was nice to have a commendation and a feeling that my work really was appreciated.

But what about my co-workers? Every one of them had huddled under heavy blankets comforting their patients while powerful, noisy, terrifying tools ripped the wrecked car apart so the patient could be safely removed. Every one of them had treated fire victims – often in closer proximity to the fire than is recommended. Every one of them had walked into patients' homes not knowing what they would find on the other side of the door. Every one of them had responded to accidents wondering if the first clue of a hazardous material leak would come when the second responding unit found their bodies unconscious or dead on the pavement.

And what about the firemen? Memories of firemen literally running through a wall of flames to reach the screaming children on the other side jumped into my mind. Memories of a fireman slipping on an icy rooftop and plunging three stories to his death haunted me.

What about the policemen? One officer had disarmed a psychiatric patient I had been unsuccessfully trying to deal with. Others had controlled unruly crowds allowing me to perform my tasks unhampered. On more than one occasion a policeman had placed his body between mine and the body of a threatening adversary.

What about the plethora of military heroes or the citizen who apprehends a purse-snatcher on the street? What about the child who pauses to get her younger sibling before leaving her burning home? What about the teachers who could easily get a much more lucrative job in the corporate world but instead dedicate themselves to teaching our children for the future benefit of mankind?

Don't all of these people deserve citations and a whole lot more?

The public perception of heroes is that they are super-human extraordinary people. Are they?

If you count all the people who routinely perform these duties you will find they number in the millions. Just by the sheer numbers these people become defined as ordinary.

Does this mean the ordinary person is a hero? If you look deep enough you will find the answer.

Someone once proclaimed there are no heroes – only ordinary people reacting to extraordinary circumstances.

27. Double Jeopardy

It wasn't fair. It wasn't supposed to happen like this.

We knew Clarence was in trouble before we could even see him. We heard the fluid gurgling in his lungs with every gasping respiration from the hallway as we approached his room. He had one of the worst cases of acute pulmonary edema I had ever seen.

As we drew closer I could see the frothy sputum spewing from his mouth with every exhalation. His extremities were swollen to twice their normal size and his blood pressure was sky high.

Clarence was scared. He knew he was going to die. He told Sylvia and I so. He was one of those patients.

I was searching frantically for a vein to start an IV, but his swollen extremities made them almost impossible to find. I was having trouble and precious time was slipping away. Sylvia managed to get one started for me.

He stopped breathing. Sylvia starting ventilating him, first with mouth to mouth resuscitation, then with the bag mask and oxygen I handed her.

I started to get my equipment to pass an endotracheal tube down into his lungs, but before I had a chance to intubate him, Sylvia yelled that he was in cardiac arrest.

A glance at the monitor told me that he was in electro-mechanical dissociation. His heart still had organized electrical activity, but the muscle had been weakened by the lack of oxygen to the point where it could no longer pump effectively.

Sylvia started CPR while I intubated him. With a patent airway in place we could oxygenate his lungs better.

I pushed some sodium bicarbonate through the IV to combat the acidosis I knew was building up in his blood.

His pulse returned and Clarence started breathing on his own again. Sylvia continued to assist his respirations with the bag mask and oxygen. His blood pressure was sky-high again and his lungs were still filled with fluid, but it was amazing we had gotten this far with a patient in his condition.

I contacted the hospital. Dr. Torres was on. He hesitated a second and then ordered me to give morphine and lasix IV push.

It was a very aggressive order and I was uncertain of it. It had sounded like Dr. Torres was uncertain of it too.

You don't usually give morphine to unconscious patients, especially right after a cardiac arrest. His blood pressure was still high and his pulse was fast, so they would be okay. Clarence was still intubated so we could easily breathe for him if the morphine knocked out his respirations.

The morphine would help clear the fluid out of his lungs and he didn't have time to wait for the Lasix. Lasix would take 20 minutes to take effect. By then Clarence would be dead.

Dr. Torres was one of our better doctors.

Besides, there really was no choice. There was nothing else I could do and doing nothing would be fatal.

I pushed the morphine through Clarence's veins and followed it with the Lasix.

In a couple of minutes Clarence started to move a little bit and then awoke with a start. I couldn't believe it. Ten minutes ago I wouldn't have given one in a thousand odds on his life but now I was witnessing a miracle.

And as I watched, paralyzed by awe for just a second or two, Clarence reached up and yanked his endotracheal tube out. As he did that the IV pulled out of his vein.

What a stupid fool I was. I should have anticipated and tied his hands down.

Clarence was talking to us once again and once more expressing his fear of dying. What he didn't know and we didn't tell his was that he already had died.

There wasn't anything more I could do for him so instead of trying to restart the troublesome IV I decided to rush him to the hospital.

Just as we reached the door, Clarence passed out again.

I looked at the EKG monitor. It was flat!

It couldn't be. I checked and double checked the leads. They were fine.

I checked for a pulse. There was no pulse. Sylvia resumed CPR while I re-intubated Clarence. Now I needed the IV but once again I had trouble with it. Once again Sylvia came to my rescue. It just wasn't my night.

I informed the hospital of what had happened and Dr. Torres ordered every cardiac arrest medication we have. I tried them all: sodium bicarbonate, epinephrine, atropine, calcium chloride, isuprel. Nothing worked.

We continued CPR enroute to the hospital but we knew the miracle had slipped between our fingers. There was only one thing left to do when we got to the hospital.

Dr. Torres made the official pronouncement of death.

We hadn't even finished restocking and cleaning the rig when a heart attack patient called for help.

Sylvia and I looked at each other. We really weren't up to it, but there wasn't any choice.

28. Wouldn't It Be Nice?

It wasn't pretty but it worked and that's all any of us can hope for.

Frieda was on the floor when we got to her. She was just starting to turn blue as she took a final gasping agonal breath. She was 67-years-old and 200 pounds.

Ben started CPR while I took out the EKG paddles to do a "quick look" at her heart's EKG. Frieda was in ventricular fibrillation, a rapid and chaotic electrical pattern which leaves the heart quivering like a sack of wriggling worms instead of pumping effectively. It is the most common cause of death in heart patients.

I charged the defibrillator and yelled "clear". Ben jumped back out of the way, knowing that if he accidentally received part of the electrical shock I was preparing to administer it could put him in cardiac arrest, too. I've never been any good at doing CPR on two patients simultaneously.

I pressed the defibrillator paddles down firmly on the protective gel pads I had placed on Frieda's chest; one just below the right collarbone, the other below her left breast and off to the side.

I squeezed the two discharge buttons, sending a shock of 400 joules traveling through Frieda's heart. It was intended to override and stop the ventricular fibrillations, allowing the natural rhythm to return.

Somehow, part of the shock must have backed up into my EKG monitor because it suddenly stopped working. I tried using the cables with the round sticky disc electrodes instead of the paddle electrodes, but they didn't work either.

A pulse check told us Frieda was still in cardiac arrest, but I had no idea what the electrical rhythm was. We restarted CPR.

I radioed in for another unit to be sent from the station, signal 10.

While waiting for the second EKG, I prepared to intubate Freida. When I put my laryngoscope into her mouth to visualize her vocal cords, she gagged and started to breathe. Another pulse check told us her heart was beating once again.

After starting the IV, I gave some sodium bicarbonate – the only drug I could give safely without knowing what her rhythm was.

When the backup unit arrived, I discovered Frieda was in atrial flutter. I could safely give lidocaine to keep her from returning to ventricular fibrillation again. I gave a 100 milligram lidocaine bolus through the IV and followed it with a continuous lidocaine drip to maintain a therapeutic level of the drug.

While giving report to the hospital, Frieda's heart converted to sinus bradycardia (a slightly slower than normal rhythm), with frequent PVC's (despite the lidocaine we had given).

The ER doctor ordered atropine which increased Frieda's heart rate and eliminated the PVC's.

She was now in normal sinus rhythm. Her pupils were reacting to light, she was breathing on her own, and her blood pressure was good.

We exchanged our nearly empty oxygen cylinder for a fresh one and took Frieda out to the ambulance.

After several weeks in the hospital Frieda was discharged and eventually returned to work as a medical receptionist.

Wouldn't it be nice if all our calls could end this way?

29. Politics

At last something was being done. I was working for a county ambulance service that was divided into 3 districts, each with a separate governing board and administrator. The morale at District 3 where I had worked during the last three years had been rock bottom. All we had ever asked for was a good, effective administrator.

All we had ever received were politicians, appointed by their own governing board to serve as part time administrators. These people had no experience in either the medical field or in any type of emergency service.

No wonder things were falling apart. It seems incredible that this could have been allowed to happen. Yet, as any EMT can tell you, it's still happening today.

I suppose the underlying root of the problem is entwined in the insurance and the Medicare and Medicaid programs. You see, they don't like to pay bills. It might subtract from the number of Super Bowl commercials they can buy.

Advanced life support ambulances save lives. They also shorten hospital stays and decrease disability time. In short, they save insurance companies LOTS of money by decreasing their payments on life, medical, and disability insurance.

Advanced life support ambulances also cost money. Adding $50-75,000 worth of equipment to each $50,000 ambulance and keeping it staffed with a minimum crew of two, 24 hours/day, 7days/week is not cheap. But the savings afforded the insurance companies are worth many times the paltry sums they pay for an ambulance run. These paltry reimbursements don't come close to paying the true cost of the service.

As a result, most advanced life support emergency services are heavily funded with tax dollars. Along with tax dollars comes politicians.

It wouldn't be so bad if they gave us our yearly allotment with a warning that they were going to check up on us. They could check with our medical director to make sure our patients were still receiving proper treatment. They could mail out questionnaires to our patients with their bills to determine if we were providing swift, courteous, and satisfactory service. They could oversee our finances to make sure the tax money they gave us was being used appropriately.

These things would allow them to confirm that the public's money is being well spent. This is not only their right; it is their obligation. None of us have any quarrel with this.

We do object when a politician pays himself tax money to administer the day-to-day operations of an ambulance service which he knows nothing about. Just as bad is when a political board concerns themselves with the details of the operation to the point where the administrator is turned into a figurehead.

This is not only a waste of taxpayers' money. It is also a danger to the public and a betrayal of their trust.

Our last part time political administrator had been forced to resign for reasons hidden in a veil of secrecy. We were promised that our next administrator would be a full time medical professional. We adopted a cautious wait and see attitude.

Our hopes dimmed when an interim board of four politicians was appointed to oversee the day-to-day operations.

The little morale that was left was dashed when two of these people were subsequently appointed permanent part time co-administrators.

A letter was composed objecting to this latest deceit and abandonment of common sense. It was signed by virtually all members of the service and submitted to these co-administrators by our shift captains. It was all kept within channels and was not publicized at that point.

For the next week everyone's spirits were sky-high. Surely a unanimous appeal based on common sense issues would have considerable influence on the board.

We were all stunned when we were informed that our shift captains had been fired. No official reason was given and the subject was not open to discussion. I guess there wasn't really anything to discuss anyway.

I resigned the following day and have never returned to full time ambulance service. They had not only destroyed what little leadership was left; they had also fired three of our best and most experienced working crew members. This action severely decreased the quality of our service and also left us very short-staffed. Their total lack of concern for the public's welfare was astounding.

After resigning I took my case to the public. What followed was one of the saddest commentaries on the American political system I have ever witnessed.

Over 1,000 residents of our small town signed a petition requesting either re-instatement of the shift captains or justification for the board's action. They got neither.

Letters to the editor appeared daily for months in support of the shift captains in both of our daily local newspapers to no avail.

The board's usually deserted meeting room was packed to overflowing with an angry crowd of voters demanding justice. They received none.

Now, more than four years later, the lawsuit filed by the shift captains is still waiting to see its first day in court.

The effect on me remains devastating. I've seen a few ambulance services get along very well with their governing boards. Even these places, however, leave me fearful. You can see a lot of politicians in a 30 year career and any one of them could end it for you. Maybe it isn't a career at all.

Score a big one for the bad guys.

30. Community Spirit

While District 3 was in controversy, District 1 and District 2, were providing excellent ambulance services under the supervision of full time professional administrators and administrative boards with a "hands off" policy. These three district services combined gave advanced life support care to the entire county.

The county commissioners had been expressing a desire to take over control of all three ambulance services for some time. The fiasco at District 3 gave them the opportunity to try to do just that.

They decided to abolish the three area services and establish one county-wide service. This new service would operate under a county EMS commission whose members would all be appointed by the commissioners. A full time professional administrator would be hired who would serve "at the pleasure" of the county commissioners.

It didn't sound like a way to end politics in EMS and it wasn't.

What followed was a controversy that made District 3's problems pale by comparison. It continues to this day.

District 1 and District 2 decided they didn't like being abolished and decided to continue service without the commissioners' support.

District 1 had an alternate source of funding and managed to pull through in pretty good shape. District 2, however, had problems.

The commissioners knew District 1 could survive without their support. They also knew a county ambulance would sit idle there. The people had grown to respect their local service and had no reason to use a different one.

District 2 had the same support and trust of the people, but was financially vulnerable. The commissioners decided to leave District 1 without county service (even though they were paying for it through taxes) and to compete with District 2.

This was a major miscalculation on their part which they have still not admitted and for which the taxpayers of the county are still paying.

The commissioners failed to take into account the close ties that had developed and the resolve of the District 2 board, administrator, employees, and the public.

District 2 became a semi-volunteer service, offering only substandard pay to its employees. The administrator, Ryan, continued his duties without any compensation. Even so, it would have all fallen apart without an extraordinary amount of support from the public.

I have worked for many different types of ambulance services in many different areas. I have enjoyed the support of the public in all of these places throughout my career. When I started working part-time for District 2, however, I found a level of support, enthusiasm, and love from the public that I had never experienced anywhere else.

The residents of the small communities served by District 2 continue to call their own semi-volunteer service in their time of need. The county ambulance still sits idle.

Despite being forced to pay for a county ambulance they will not use, these people fund District 2 through fund raising efforts, donations, and a membership program. They are truly marvelous.

The commissioners meanwhile have floundered along without any clear direction, continuing to waste taxpayers' money.

One of their strongest arguments for the attempted takeover was to save costs. Yet, the EMS budget was virtually the same after the takeover despite the fact they weren't providing service to Area I and were only providing rare backup service in Area II.

It is unfortunate District 2 does not have the financial resources to offer a true EMS career opportunity. Also, there is no guarantee that what happened at District 3 and at the present county system couldn't happen to District 2 someday too.

Despite these drawbacks, the public appreciation in District 2, combined with the unique ability of the governing board to differentiate between regulating and interfering, have resulted in greater satisfaction than I have ever found anywhere else.

31. Don't Dare Look

I was studying the 15-month-old body that was lying lifeless in my arm. I had taken her from her father and started CPR. At the same time I was examining her to the point where after only 30 seconds I knew her body better than her parents did.

I knew her approximate size and weight. The exact color of her skin had been noted and I was watching it change as her cyanosis lessened as we performed CPR.

The neck was soft and pliable as it should be, not rigid as you might find with meningitis.

A quick inspection and palpitation had failed to find any sign of external trauma or internal hemorrhage.

There was no swelling in the facial area and my puffs of air were moving into her lungs easily – no airway obstruction or allergic reaction.

I knew exactly how compliant her rib cage was and had gauged the exact amount of pressure necessary to compress her sternum about one inch for CPR.

I peered into her eyes hoping to find some slight reaction in them to my penlight. There was none.

All of these things I had observed and noted within the first 30 seconds – but I hadn't really seen her. Not yet. I didn't dare. I never really look at my patients until the run is over.

It wasn't anyone's fault. The babysitter had dutifully put her to bed. Her parents checked her when they got home and found her this way. There had been no warning to either the babysitter or the parents.

They knew it was too late. I knew it too. But even if there was only one chance in a thousand, I had to make sure.

I also knew the probable cause was SIDS (Sudden Infant Death Syndrome) – I continued CPR enroute to the hospital. There the doctor worked on her for another hour. Finally, we were all forced to accept the inevitable. She was dead.

I looked at her for the first time. She looked strikingly similar to my own 15-month-old daughter.

The rest of the night dragged on forever. In the morning when my shift was finally over, I raced home to be with my daughter, Katy.

I spent the next few days holding, hugging, and kissing Katy. Even at her young age the look in her eyes told me she thought her Daddy had gone crazy. She didn't understand why I wouldn't let go of her.

I hope she never has to understand.

32. The Other Side Of The Coin

"Ben," Fran called to her 17-year-old son. "Ben, I need some help, come here."

Her husband was at work and she needed help carrying some heavy boxes downstairs to the basement.

"Ben, where are you?"

In just a few short months Ben would be leaving for college and she would only see him on weekends. Of course, when she considered how much she sees of him now she wasn't sure how much of a difference it would make.

"Ben, answer me," she yelled angrily. He was still living at home and could certainly help with a few minor household chores. She went in search of him.

"Oh my God, Ben what's wrong?" Fran screamed seeing her son lying on the floor.

There was no answer. He was unconscious. It looked like he was breathing, but she wasn't sure.

"What should I do," she wondered frantically. She raced to the phone and looked up their doctor's number.

"Dr. Evan's answering service, please hold."

"Don't put me on hold," she started to yell but she heard the click before the first word was out. She fidgeted nervously wondering if her son was still alive.

"Thank you for holding, can I help you?"

"Yes," Fran shouted. "I need to speak to Dr. Evans right away."

"I'm sorry, Dr. Evans doesn't have office hours today. You'll have to call back tomorrow."

"This is an emergency. My son is sick and I need the doctor right now."

"Ma'am, if this is an emergency, then Dr. Evans suggests you go to the nearest emergency room," said the girl.

"I just told you my son is sick," Fran yelled. "He's unconscious and I can't get him to the hospital. My husband's at work. I don't even know if he's alive and ---"

"Ma'am, it sounds to me like you should call an ambulance," she interrupted.

"Alright, what's their number?" Fran inquired.

"I don't know ma'am. That depends on where you live."

"I live in Charleston," Fran screamed in frustration. "What's the number for the Charleston ambulance?"

"I really don't know. You'll have to look it up."

Fran slammed the receiver down and grabbed the phone book again.

First she looked in the white pages under "Charleston, City of". She found the police department and the fire department, but no ambulance. Did the fire department or police department run the ambulance? Fran didn't know.

She turned to the yellow pages and looked under "Ambulance". There was a county service, but she didn't know if they covered the entire county or just the unincorporated areas.

There were three ambulance companies listed in the book located in Charleston. Their ads all talked about transferring patients – but they also said they were staffed by emergency medical technicians. Did they handle emergencies or didn't they?

By now she was in tears as she called the telephone operator for help.

"I need an ambulance right now," Fran told her.

"Which ambulance service do you want?" the operator inquired.

"I don't know, any one. I just need one right away," Fran cried.

"Where are you calling from?"

"Charleston," Fran replied.

"Okay, hold on. I'll connect you with the Charleston Police Department," the operator said.

Click, click.

"Charleston Police, is this an emergency?" a business – like voice asked.

"Yes, I need an ambulance right away," she repeated for seemingly the umpteenth time.

"What's your address?" the officer asked.

"1417 Coldwater Drive," Fran answered.

"You should have called the county ambulance service directly, but I'll take the information and call them for you. I need your name, a description of your house, the nature of the problem, and your phone number."

"I don't have time," Fran shouted angrily. "My son's dying and I have to go check on him."

She slammed down the receiver and ran back to her son in tears. These people were supposed to be professionals. Why were they wasting time asking stupid questions? When this was all over, she would see to it they got a piece of her mind.

Ben still looked the same. She wasn't sure if he was alive or not. Should she pound on his chest or blow into his mouth like she had seen them do on TV? Fran didn't know. Why didn't the police give her instructions?

What was taking so long? An ambulance should be quick. They're supposed to save lives.

Finally Fran heard the siren off in the distance. It was slowly getting louder, but it was taking an agonizingly long time. She bet they weren't even doing the speed limit.

She watched out the window as they drove right past the house.

"What's wrong with them?" Fran screamed, cursing them under her breath. She knew the mailbox didn't have the house number on it. No one around here had a number on their box. But their name was on it. Weren't they looking?

She left her dying son and ran outside in time to see them returning from the other direction driving very slowly. She tried to wave them down.

When they spotted her they came roaring into the driveway, turning almost on two wheels, and came to a screeching stop; obviously trying to impress her.

"What's the problem?" one of them asked as he jumped out.

"Follow me," Fran yelled angrily, running inside.

159

She reached her son, turned around, and discovered she was alone. Where were they?

In a little while they came in carrying a bunch of kits and boxes. There was a green tank with a gauge on it that looked like oxygen. Another one Fran recognized from TV. It was one of those machines with a screen on it and the paddles they use to "zap" you. She hoped they wouldn't zap Ben. Those things even made dead people jump. There was another box marked "AIRWAY" and one marked "PEDS".

The medic who seemed to be in charge turned to his partner and said, "Take out the pediatrics kit and bring in the med box."

"Why had they brought in a pediatric kit?" Fran wondered. Another waste of time.

Suddenly she realized they hadn't brought a stretcher in.

"Where's the stretcher?" she demanded.

"We have to examine and treat your son first," was the reply.

Why were they being so difficult?

"Stop wasting time and get him to the hospital," Fran screamed. "You're not doctors."

"We're working under written orders of the emergency room physicians and carrying out their instructions to the letter," replied the medic in charge.

The entire time he continued examining Ben, his eyes never leaving Fran's son as he spoke to her. He did look like he knew what he was doing. Fran just wished she could be sure.

"Does Ben have any medical problems like high blood pressure, diabetes, epilepsy, asthma, or anything else you can think of?" the other medic asked her.

"No," Fran answered. "He's usually as healthy as a horse."

"Does he take any medication?"

"No," she answered.

"Has he been feeling okay lately and has he been eating normally?"

"Well, he has been feeling a bit funny lately," she replied. "Nothing specific, but I made a doctor's appointment for next week. I wanted him to have a good physical before going away to college. As for eating, he's been eating more than ever. Mostly junk food."

The medic had turned Ben onto his side and placed a funny looking curved white tube into his mouth. The oxygen mask was in place and he was getting ready to start an IV.

Fran had always been squeamish about needles so she turned her head so she wouldn't see. Her curiosity got the better of her, however, and she peeked to see how much it was hurting Ben.

The panic that had started to subside was returning again. Bed didn't even flinch.

"Is he dead?" Fran asked hesitantly. She was afraid to hear the answer.

"No, he isn't," the medic reassured her while placing a drop of blood from the IV on a little plastic stick. "His vitals are fine right now and I'm trying to find out why he's unconscious."

He reached into the med box his partner has brought in and withdrew a blue box. It was larger than most of the others Fran saw in the kit. When he opened it she saw why. She was shocked to see him take out the biggest needle and syringe she had ever seen.

"Do you have to stick him with that?" Fran asked.

"No," the medic answered. "I'm going to inject this through his IV."

Fran didn't want to interrupt him but she was dying to know what it was.

"It's kind of sugar water," was the reply.

"He's not diabetic," Fran said with alarm.

"It's okay," the medic assured her. "Maybe he is a diabetic now and that's why he hasn't been feeling well. Also, you don't have to be a diabetic to have low blood sugar. Anyway, even if that isn't the problem, this stuff won't do any harm."

How did he become so good at never breaking his concentration or letting his eyes wander from his work while answering her questions at the same time, Fran wondered.

He pushed the needle into the IV tubing and injected it slowly.

Just seconds after he finished, Fran saw Ben start to move. The medic quickly withdrew the curved white tube from Ben's mouth.

Fran wanted to jump for joy but she was afraid to; still uncertain of what the final outcome might be.

The medic was taking vitals again while his partner went outside. He returned with a stretcher. They lifted Ben onto the stretcher and strapped him in. Then he reached into the kit and took out another big blue box. He gave it the same way he had the first time.

This time Ben's eyes opened. He looked around in alarm and asked, "Where am I? What happened?"

"You're okay," answered the medic. "You passed out but you're doing fine now. Here's your mom."

"Can I touch him?" Fran asked, barely able to restrain herself.

"Sure," replied the medic smiling and looking at her for the first time. "Just be careful with the IV."

She bent over and kissed him. "I was so afraid you were going to die," she told him.

Then they took him out to the ambulance. They told Fran she had to ride up front and wear the seat belt. On the way in she could hear the medic in charge reporting to the hospital from a radio in the back.

Fran was afraid she would get sick riding in front during a wild ambulance ride, but it wasn't really that wild or fast. She remembered her anger at them taking so long to get to Ben, but she was so happy right now that it didn't matter.

When she called her husband Ken from the hospital and told him what happened, he left work immediately and rushed right over. Fran was still in the waiting room when he got there. She had a thousand things to tell him and she didn't know where to begin.

Fran started relaying her story while they anxiously waited to hear from the doctor.

She told him about the trouble she had finding the right phone number. "We have to make a list of all of the emergency numbers and keep it by the phone," she told him.

Her husband nodded his agreement. "We'll keep a list by each of the phones," he added.

"That police dispatcher really asked some stupid questions," Fran said. "Who cares what my name is or what our house looks like in an emer---,". She stopped in mid-sentence. Fran suddenly realized why the ambulance had driven past their house the first time. Visions of the box with "PEDS" on it came to her as she heard herself telling the dispatcher her son was sick. She remembered cursing him for not giving her instructions a few short seconds after she hung up on him.

Fran felt guilty for acting so panicked and foolish.

"But it really did take them an awful long time to get there," she told Ken.

Ken looked at her and frowned. "When did all this happen?"

Fran remembered looking at the clock just before she found Ben. It was 5 o'clock and she would have to start getting supper ready. That's why she had wanted him to help with those heavy boxes.

Her husband looked perplexed. "It's only 6:15 now," he pointed out. "It took me at least 25 minutes to get here."

Fran checked her watch. She couldn't believe it, but he was right. She had been at the hospital for a few minutes before calling Ken. Was it possible all this had occurred in less than an hour?

A nurse finally told them they could see Ben. He looked fine and Fran could see the relief on Ken's face when he finally got to see his son.

The ER doctor wanted to admit him for tests. Ken and Fran agreed.

A few days later they met with their family doctor for instructions just before he discharged Ben.

He ended by saying, "If you follow these instructions we shouldn't have to save Ben's life anymore."

"Could he really have died?" Fran asked with a lump in her throat.

"Definitely," replied Dr. Evans.

As they drove home Fran relived the scene of a few days earlier once again.

"We ought to send a thank you note to those medics," she said.

"Do you know their names?" Ken asked.

"No, I don't. They left the emergency room for another call before I could find out," Fran answered.

"I don't know their names either," said Ben.

"Well how would you address it then?" asked Ken.

"I don't know."

33. More Winter Fun

Chicago and its neighboring areas are notorious for harsh winters and this one was no exception.

As I drove carefully on icy roads through the snow-blanketed farm land I couldn't help thinking of an Arctic wasteland. The temperature of -10 $^\circ$ F with a wind chill factor of -60 $^\circ$ F did little to change my mind.

I was on my way to work at a rural ambulance station; the one where a strong wind would blow out a lit match in the center of the building.

I already knew what to expect when I got there. Inevitably we were going to be called out on an auto accident. There was no use worrying about it. It was useless to hope for anything else. No amount of wishful thinking could change our fate. We were going to get an auto accident.

It was a simple and inescapable law of nature. The colder and nastier the weather, the more certain it is you will get called out for an auto accident.

If I could find some sucker to bet against this principle, I'd be a millionaire; but no one is that big a sucker.

This winter was the worst since I moved here three years ago. We had already recorded temperatures of -27°F with a wind chill factor of -95°F. In comparison, I guess you would have to consider this day as "mild". Nevertheless, it was cold enough to guarantee an auto accident.

I groped into my deep coat pockets, past my work gloves and my ski gloves, to make sure I had my jar of Vaseline. Vaseline smeared over my face would help protect me from frostbite if I was stuck outside for a long time. That's what I was hoping, anyway.

Weather like this presents us with numerous challenges. Not the least of these is avoiding frostbite, pneumonia, hypothermia, and just plain freezing to death ourselves. For our patients it's even worse.

Do we risk moving a potential spinal injury patient without taking time for proper immobilization to get him out of the cold? This could result in permanent paralysis. The alternative is to take the time to properly immobilize the spine and in the process preserve it as well in a human ice cube – all for a patient who might not have any spinal injury anyway.

If you've ever noticed how large your veins get when you're washing dishes in hot water, you've probably realized veins like warmth. Conversely, veins hate cold. What are the chances of starting an IV in veins so cold and contracted, they can't even be seen? Especially when my hands are shaking so bad from the cold that I couldn't hit the side of a barn?

How fast dare we drive on icy roads to reach a patient who is dying?

How many of the signs that we see in our patient are from the cold and not the injury?

How many signs and symptoms from the injury are masked by the cold?

The list goes on and on.

There's only one thing I like about winter. Every winter I like the fact that I'm not a fireman.

I've seen too many living sheets of ice with fire coats underneath to ever want to be a fireman in the winter. They get sprayed with the water and are instantly converted to giant human ice pops. They are literally covered with ice from head to foot; hair, skin, clothes and all. I've seen this happen at several major fire scenes even in New Jersey; and back there the temperatures seldom dropped below a balmy 0°F.

Anyway, on this day Carlos would wait until 3:00 am before running his van off the road and into a tree. His head struck the windshield with enough force to pop it out. At the same time the roof buckled, coming down behind his head and trapping him there with his head protruding through where the windshield had once been. The most amazing thing was despite all of this, he had no obvious major injuries.

There was no way I was going to cut his coat off out there to get a blood pressure and an examination of his torso. He was conscious and alert with strong pulses and no apparent distress. That was good enough for me.

We covered him with blankets and went to work tearing what was left of his van apart. To maintain good spinal immobilization we had to cut the roof and peel it back out of the way before taking Carlos out.

It seemed to take hours, though it didn't of course. Throughout it all Carlos remained stable and was even in pretty good spirits.

We finally managed to free him. We applied the cervical collar and short spineboard and slid him out of the van onto a long spineboard. We rushed inside for the warmth of the ambulance.

Once there I started cutting off his clothes while my partner reached for a blood pressure cuff.

I heard a crash as it hit the floor and turned to see the gauge of the blood pressure cuff lying in pieces on the floor. Fingers numb from the cold are not very dexterous.

I continued my examination while my partner got our second blood pressure cuff (also our last blood pressure cuff). Everything seemed fine until my partner called out a blood pressure reading of 60/20.

I looked at Carlos. Then I looked at my partner. It couldn't be. Anyone with a blood pressure that low would be showing obvious signs of shock. I checked the blood pressure myself and got the same reading.

We put the Medical Anti-Shock Trousers on Carlos but I didn't inflate them yet. I still wasn't convinced. With a blood pressure of 60/20 I shouldn't have been able to feel a radial pulse – but the pulse was still strong. It should have been very rapid, attempting to compensate for the low blood pressure, but it wasn't.

I knew I should start at least one IV just in case and proceeded to get one set up.

When I looked at his arms, however, there wasn't a vein in sight. I took out a needle and prepared to make a "blind stick" into an area I knew should contain a vein. My hands were still shaking so bad from the cold that I realized I would be lucky to hit his arm with the needle. There was virtually no chance of hitting a vein.

I put the needle down and examined Carlos again. He was still conscious, alert and relaxed. His skin was still cold from being outside, but it was dry, not clammy as it should be from shock. Carlos was breathing easily and his lung sounds were clear and equal bilaterally. There was no bruising, swelling, or tenderness to the chest, abdomen, or thighs. Carlos still had no complaints other than the cold and his pulses were still strong.

There was no way he needed an IV. The blood pressure cuff had to be wrong.

We started driving to the hospital while I called in my report. It took a lot of talking to dissuade the ER doctor from ordering me to attempt an IV.

When we got to the hospital Carlos and his blood pressure were fine. Our blood pressure cuff, however, was not feeling too well. A check revealed that it was off by 50 mm Hg.

My next shift was three days later and by then I had just barely warmed up enough to go out and do it all over again.

34. Trauma!

I do not believe in a lot of laws, regulations, and governmental influence. Basically I believe no law should be passed until it is proved to have a distinct and clear-cut advantage to the general population or to protect the rights of individuals.

Avoiding the death of millions of people is a distinct clear-cut advantage.

I have been called to the scene of thousands of auto accidents. Too many of them have been fatal.

I don't need any government statistic to tell me the factors involved in lethal auto accidents. I have my own. There are three factors and almost all accidents involving a fatality have all three of these factors present:

1. Speed
2. Not using seatbelts
3. Alcohol

If you remove any of these three factors, most of the fatal accidents I've seen wouldn't have been fatal. Many of them wouldn't have occurred at all.

Calls that come in shortly after the closing time of the local bars are always trouble. You know that even before the phone rings a second time. That's when this call came in.

I responded with everything I had; one advanced life support ambulance, one basic life support ambulance, and the fire department. It wasn't enough.

The accident scene was a rural country road. Only one car was involved. Pieces of that car were lying everywhere. Several small trees had been sheared off. What was left of the front end of the car was wrapped around a large tree.

Inside the car were two college girls home for the weekend.

One was lying in a twisted heap on the floor in front. She was moaning and moving a bit but she was unconscious.

The other girl had been thrown backward. She was draped face up over the back of the front seat with her head and shoulders in the back.

A nurse had happened across the scene and was in the back seat doing mouth-to-mouth resuscitation on the bloodied face of the second girl. She informed me that just seconds ago she had lost the girl's pulse.

I radioed our dispatcher to send an additional advanced life support unit from the country ambulance service. Then I grabbed the girl in cardiac arrest and dragged her out of the car supporting her head and neck the best I could. She didn't have time to wait for cervical collars and spineboards.

One of my crew members and the nurse stayed with me. I assigned the rest of my crew and the fire department to take care of the other girl still inside the car pending arrival of the second paramedic unit.

I suctioned blood out of my patient's mouth and took over CPR using the jaw thrust maneuver to open the airway while my partner got an esophageal obturator airway (EOA) for me to insert. At the time, the EOA was the only airway we were permitted to use for patients with potential cervical injuries. It isn't as good as an endotracheal tube, but it's better than anything else.

I inserted the EOA and we started ventilating her through it with supplemental oxygen.

We applied and inflated the MAST while placing her on a long spineboard at the same time. I inserted two large bore intravenous lines while racing to the hospital with her.

My radio report was short and to the point.

"We are enroute with a Class IV Trauma Alert patient in full arrest. Obvious head and neck injuries present. You will be contacted by Rescue 3 regarding a second patient at the scene who was still alive. Our ETA is 15 minutes." There was no time to elaborate and nothing else was needed.

They continued working on her in the emergency room, but there really hadn't been any chance from the beginning.

In the meantime, I was getting funny looks from a lot of people. I didn't know why until I got a glimpse of myself in the mirror. My face was covered with the girl's blood from doing mouth-to-mouth resuscitation on her.

Within minutes the other ambulance brought the second girl in. She was critical but she was still alive. She was also drunk. She was the driver. She survived.

I fully support the enactment and strict enforcement of all laws related to speed limits, seat belt usage, and drunk driving. It's time for the killing to stop.

35. Personally Speaking

By now you probably have a pretty good idea of what the professional life of a medic is like. But what about the personal life?

As you have seen, the job we do is rooted in instability. We soon learn not to count on anything but ourselves and our partner. In my personal life I look for a level of stability that matches the level of instability I deal with on my job.

Let's face it, if we didn't have stability at some point in our lives, there wouldn't be any medics in the field. We'd all be in insane asylums.

This is not to say that the home life of a medic is completely normal. We tend to have some idiosyncrasies which border on fanaticism.

You cannot fit anything into the trunk of a medic's car. This is because we all carry our own personal first aid kits that just barely fit into the trunk. Whenever I happen across an accident I'm always careful of whom I ask to run to my car to get my kit. If I don't pick someone strong enough, they'll never make it back.

A three piece suit is not the ideal uniform for a medic, but if that's what I'm wearing when I come across an accident, that becomes my uniform. I must admit, however, that mud, blood, and vomitus don't do much to help the appearance of a suit.

If you walked into my house you might be surprised to see the ceilings plastered with smoke detectors. My wife's objection did not deter me from putting one in the kitchen where it goes off every night at suppertime. "The kitchen is a common source of fire," I argued. "Besides, at least we know it's working".

I would also bet you couldn't find a closet or cabinet door to open that doesn't have a fire extinguisher behind it. I'm not talking about the little ones capable of extinguishing a cigarette. Mine range in size from six to ten pounds.

Those of you who are parents are familiar with being awakened in the middle of the night by your crying children. Not me. When they stop crying I become alarmed and go to check on them. What caused them to stop? Since my wife is not as impervious to their screams as I am, she ends up with more than her share of interrupted sleep. This pattern became evident with the birth of our daughter, Katy, and has since re-emerged with the birth of our son, David.

A good deal of our income is spent on every book and journal I can find related to emergency medicine.

Where can you find a woman who can provide the extreme stability I require even in the face of all of these peculiarities?

She has to tolerate long periods of being away from home – and then being too exhausted to do anything but sleep when I finally get home.

She has to have the trust to allow me to sleep overnight with another woman when the ambulance schedule calls for it.

She has to understand the many moods I bring home from the job with me. She must know when to comfort, when to talk, and when to leave me alone.

She has to be able to listen to my stories of blood and guts when I need to talk, without running out of the room sick.

She has to approve of a level of dedication to my work which drastically interferes with our family life; knowing at the same time that the usual financial rewards for such dedication do not exist in this job.

Where can you find a person like this?

You can't. There can be only one in the whole world. Her name is Teresa. She's mine, and you can't have her.

36. Reflections

By most standards fourteen years is a very short career. In EMS, fourteen years is forever. It has been a long, hard, and very rewarding career. I have had experiences which I wouldn't trade for anything and I can't help believing that even the tough calls contributed immensely to my development.

As I look back now, I wonder how much longer it will last. I feel like a professional athlete who is near the end of his career but too much in love to let go.

As new skills and procedures are implemented, however, I find it increasingly difficult to keep up with them on a part time basis.

I can't help thinking that I have a couple good seasons left in me – but I pray that either I will recognize when the time has come or that someone else will tell me.

EMS has been the newest and fastest growing medical profession in recent times. The past three decades have witnessed the transformation of ambulance personnel from race car drivers to highly trained medical technicians who are so specialized that some of the skills they routinely perform are things that many doctors haven't done since they attended medical school.

The technical and medical advances have saved and will continue to save countless number of victims of acute illness and injury – but more is needed.

I suppose it is the nature of the human animal to never be completely satisfied, to want just a little bit more. I am no exception.

If I had a wish list, at the top of my list would be the wish that I could have continued my EMS career on a full time basis. I wish I could have avoided some of the smaller near-sighted battles that plague every EMS career. I wish I could have recognized the basic underlying problems in EMS earlier and concentrated on doing something about them.

The EMS community needs professional organization now more than anything else. Organization to tackle and resolve the difficult issues facing us today. Organization to fight the intrusion of politics into medical management. Organization to take our case to the public and win their support for our proposals. What is good for us is good for the public and vice-versa.

The foundation has been laid and it is a strong one. It is built on the sweat and tears of thousands of dedicated men and women, some of whom I have had the honor of working with.

Now it is time for a change once again. It is time for EMS to mature into the strong, aggressive, cohesive profession it is capable of being.

It can no longer afford to bow at the feet of short-sighted, power-hungry politicians who would ruin everything we work for and justify their inordinate degree of power by our use of tax dollars.

It can no longer afford to gratefully acknowledge the token reimbursements tossed our way by the insurance companies in return for the vast savings rendered them.

It can no longer afford to let its medics be harassed and abused from outside sources to the point where the average career lasts less than five years.

Something must be done and this is the time to do it.

There are many tough decisions lying ahead. The past has been marked with in-house bickering and too much compromise. The future of EMS may well be more difficult than the past. But today's rookies are also much better than yesterday's rookies. They are better trained, better equipped, and better qualified than ever before.

The spark I have seen in their eyes assures me that EMS will continue to progress and the public will continue to be served.

www.ingramcontent.com/pod-product-compliance
Lightning Source LLC
Chambersburg PA
CBHW070856180526
45168CB00005B/1839